Living with Rheumatoid Arthritis

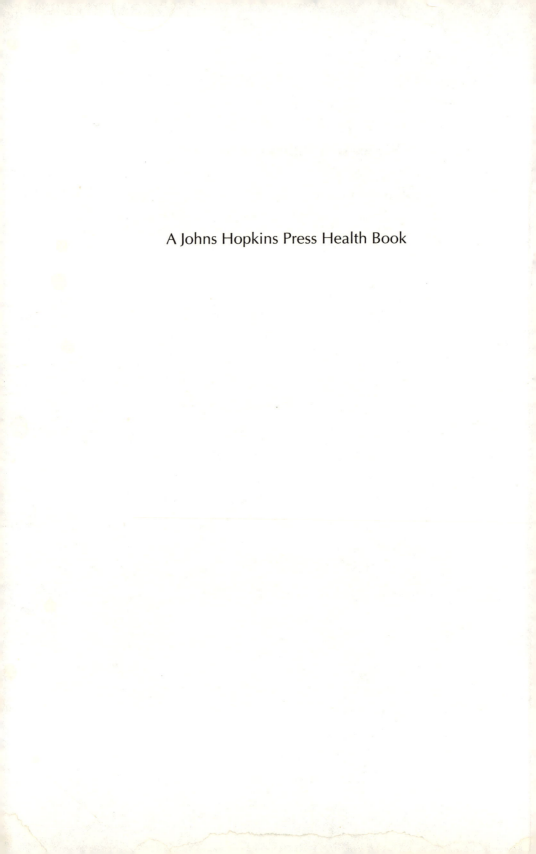

A Johns Hopkins Press Health Book

TAMMI L. SHLOTZHAUER, M.D.

JAMES L. McGUIRE, M.D.

Living with Rheumatoid Arthritis

•

SECOND EDITION

Foreword by
Carol M. Ziminski, M.D.

THE JOHNS HOPKINS UNIVERSITY PRESS

BALTIMORE AND LONDON

Note to the reader

This book is not meant to substitute for medical care of people with rheumatoid arthritis, and treatment should not be based solely on its contents. Instead, treatment must be developed in a dialogue between the individual and his or her physician. Our book has been written to help with that dialogue.

Drug dosage

The authors and publisher have exerted every effort to ensure that the selection and dosage of drugs discussed in this text accord with current recommendations and practice at the time of publication. However, in view of ongoing research, changes in governmental regulations, and the constant flow of information relating to drug therapy and drug reactions, the reader is urged to check the package insert of each drug for any change in indications and dosage and for warnings and precautions. This is particularly important when the recommended agent is a new and/or infrequently used drug.

© 1993, 2003 The Johns Hopkins University Press
All rights reserved. Published 2003
Printed in the United States of America on acid-free paper
9 8 7 6 5 4 3 2 1

Illustrations by Jacqueline Schaffer, except Figures 1, 2, and 22.
Figures 1 and 2 by Teresa Vaitkus. Figure 22 courtesy of the U.S. Department of Agriculture and the U.S. Department of Health and Human Services.

The Johns Hopkins University Press
2715 North Charles Street
Baltimore, Maryland 21218-4363
www.press.jhu.edu

Library of Congress Cataloging-in-Publication Data

Shlotzhauer, Tammi L.
Living with rheumatoid arthritis / Tammi L. Shlotzhauer, James L. McGuire;
foreword by Carol M. Ziminski.—2nd ed.
p. cm.
Includes bibliographical references and index.
ISBN 0-8018-7146-8 (hardcover: alk. paper)—ISBN 0-8018-7147-6 (pbk.: alk. paper)
1. Rheumatoid arthritis—Popular works.
[DNLM: 1. Arthritis, Rheumatoid—Popular works. WE 346 S558L 2003]
I. McGuire, James L. II. Title.
RC933.S445 2003
616.7'227—dc21
2002007593

A catalog record for this book is available from the British Library.

Contents

•

19. Surgery for Rheumatoid Arthritis   245

PART VI
Practical Matters

20. Disability, Insurance, and Other Financial Matters   253

Foreword

•

First, a story. A young girl was studying geography. She was enthralled as she learned about different places and peoples. Her heart's desire was to have a globe. For her birthday, she received a beautiful globe, and she was absolutely thrilled. She spent the entire day looking at it, studying it, and enjoying it. She even took it to bed with her, carefully cradling her prized possession. Later that evening, as her father checked on her, he gently tried to remove the globe from her arms. She awoke with a start and said, "Daddy, what are you doing with my world?"

When a person develops rheumatoid arthritis, her or his world changes, and that world can be a difficult and frightening place. Rheumatoid arthritis is a chronic disease that can adversely affect function, quality of life, and longevity. It is a leading cause of disability in the United States. Despite extensive research, we have not identified a cause, and we therefore do not have a cure. We do however, have a variety of medicines and interventions that can help manage the symptoms, and help control the disease process. In recent years, there have been significant advances in our comprehension of the processes that cause damage in rheumatoid arthritis. This has led to the development of new drugs, which have exciting potential for altering the course of the disease.

One of the most important needs of persons living with rheumatoid arthritis is education. The informed patient will have an understanding of what rheumatoid arthritis is, how it affects her or him, and how she or he can be involved in management of the disease. Family members and caregivers are also better able to provide support if they know about the disease, its potential complications, and its treatment. Patients have a better outcome when they understand more about their disease and its management.

Living with Rheumatoid Arthritis is a well-written, readable, comprehensive guide for patients who have rheumatoid arthritis, and for those who care about them and for them. The authors provide up-to-date scientific information about what rheumatoid arthritis is, and how our knowledge of the disease process has led to the development of new medicines and new approaches to management. Also included are recommendations that patients and families can implement to gain control over many aspects of the disease—physical, emotional, and practical.

This second edition has been extensively revised. It not only reviews the traditional medicines that have been used for the treatment of rheumatoid arthritis but also provides information about the newest drugs available, which can significantly improve the course of the disease. The current recommendations about prevention and treatment of osteoporosis which it offers are valuable. An important new chapter addresses alternative and complementary therapies, an area of increasing interest for many patients who may be frustrated by incomplete response to conventional medicines. An updated chapter about nutrition provides practical information about diet, vitamins, food supplements, and herbal remedies. In this computer-savvy age, there is useful advice about safely surfing the Internet. The authors also explain clinical trials, which are so important to assure the safety and effectiveness of new drugs.

I suggest that readers first scan the whole book, and then return to the chapters that are of most interest and importance to the patient, the family member, or the caregiver. The sections dealing with the mechanisms of inflammation may require more than one reading, but the reader will be rewarded with a better understanding of the disease process and the scientific basis for treatment recommendations. The chapters on exercise suggest practical answers to the questions of how much to exercise as opposed to how much to rest. The chapters on medications detail possible side effects of the various medicines and emphasize the importance of open communication between patient and physician.

Rheumatoid arthritis can present significant challenges to the patient, to family members, and to caregivers. This book will help individuals deal more positively with their disease by helping them understand what rheumatoid arthritis is and appreciate the rationale for treatment. Close cooperation among patient, family members or caregivers, physicians, and therapists can make the world a better place for the patient with rheumatoid arthritis.

Carol M. Ziminski, M.D.
Division of Rheumatology
The Johns Hopkins Medical Institutions

Preface

•

If you or someone close to you has rheumatoid arthritis, you probably have many questions about what that diagnosis means. We have written this book to answer those questions. *Living with Rheumatoid Arthritis* describes all aspects of this condition, from the physical and the emotional to the practical. We hope this book will help you not only to understand rheumatoid arthritis but also to deal constructively with the changes it may bring in your life.

This book will also let you know that you are not alone. It has been estimated that two to three million Americans have rheumatoid arthritis, with about 200,000 people being newly diagnosed each year. Worldwide, about 1 percent of the population has this condition, which affects people of all races and ethnic groups. People of all ages have rheumatoid arthritis, although it most commonly first affects people in their twenties, thirties, and forties. Three times more women than men have the condition.

Most people with rheumatoid arthritis lead highly productive, full, and satisfying lives. More than anything else, we hope that this book will provide you with the information that you need to lead as productive a life as possible.

We want to pause here to state that this book is not intended to take the place of your physician. We hope, though, that it will help you to formulate questions about your own health which you can then discuss with your doctor.

People have many different ways of coping with the knowledge that they have a chronic illness. Some people, for example, cope by denying that they have an illness; others put blind faith in their physicians and don't ask any questions or make any decisions. Others go from doctor to doctor trying anything for a cure—whether it's a proven, prescribed treatment or unconventional therapies. Some people cope by giving up and letting the illness control them: they don't follow their physician's or therapist's advice because they think nothing will help.

Studies have shown, however, that the people who cope best with a chronic illness are those who have an understanding of the disease process. This means that they learn everything they can about the illness so that they can take an active role in monitoring and caring for their own health.

What happens when you learn that you have rheumatoid arthritis? First of all, educating yourself about rheumatoid arthritis and developing realistic expectations will help you overcome your fears and decrease your anxiety. We know that fear of the unknown creates great anxiety, just as uncertainty creates stress. This is because, more often than not, our imaginations create scenarios that are much worse than the reality could ever be. The *truth,* therefore, can often be reassuring.

Second, once you understand rheumatoid arthritis, you will be able to communicate more effectively with health care professionals; the time you spend with your physician, nurse, or therapist will be more helpful to both of you. You know your body better than anyone else, and you can become an expert on *your* arthritis. Then you can work closely with your health care providers in developing a therapeutic program that is tailor-made for you and that addresses your specific needs.

Finally, what you know about your rheumatoid arthritis will help you cope more effectively with the challenges it poses. For example, you will better understand the value of medication, exercise, joint protection, and other treatments. Understanding the rationale behind each of the components of your treatment program may make you a more active participant in that program.

You can't read away your arthritis, of course, but you can play an important part in making decisions if you understand it. For all the reasons discussed above, we hope you will read on, and take a major role in mastering your arthritis.

In the first part of this book we discuss the physical aspects of rheumatoid arthritis, including changes in the joints and other parts of the body. Part II describes techniques for coping with the challenges that rheumatoid arthritis poses, and Part III introduces a series of exercises that have proven beneficial for people with this condition. In Part IV, all aspects of drug therapy are discussed. Advice about practical matters from insurance to traveling is offered in Part V. At the end of many chapters you'll find information about additional resources, including organizations and readings. At the back of the book there is a glossary of terms used in this book. Words that are defined in the glossary are set in **boldface** type at their first use in each chapter. Other important terms in the text are in *italic* type.

Acknowledgments

•

Many individuals participated in the creation of this book, and we are indebted to each of them. We especially recognize Teresa Vaitkus and Judith Nash for the countless hours they spent on the project. Their work is a complement to the text. Judith painstakingly edited the manuscript's early drafts, enhancing content, style, and comprehensibility for our non-medical readers.

We are grateful to the following medical professionals for their review of parts of the text, along with indispensable advice and comments: Robert Swezey, Janice Lambert, Ann Coulston, Paul Bergeron, Janet Price, Freddie Yee, and Elliott Ehrich. T.L.S. also thanks William Lages, Molly Fainstat, Thomas Bush, James McGuire, Elaine Lambert, and John Baum for the inspiration of their example and their teaching.

We are grateful to Jacqueline Wehmueller for her wise advice and guidance, to Anne Whitmore for her attentive copyediting, to other staff at the Johns Hopkins University Press, and to Jacqueline Schaffer for her excellent artwork.

For this second edition, I would like to acknowledge my co-author, Dr. James McGuire, who was taken from us in 1997. It was Jim's enthusiasm that carried the idea of *Living with Rheumatoid Arthritis* from dream to reality. Jim approached medicine, teaching, and life from the perspective that all things are possible. If it could be imagined, it could be accomplished. He had countless ideas, and they led to countless accomplishments. His contagious enthusiasm and undaunted optimism touched patients, students, and fellow physicians, many of whom continue to carry out his dreams.

Living with Rheumatoid Arthritis

Introduction:
Defining Rheumatoid Arthritis

•

To most people arthritis means pain and stiffness in the joints. Indeed, if you trace the word *arthritis* to its Greek roots you will discover that it means inflammation (*itis*) of the joints (*arthron*). In practice the word is used to describe more than one hundred different joint disorders, many of which are not caused by inflammation at all.

There are several forms of arthritis which *do* begin as significant inflammation in the joints, and this inflammation causes damage to the joints. Rheumatoid arthritis (RA) is a form of **inflammatory arthritis.** With RA, inflammation plays a major role in causing joint problems. This inflammation can bring about warmth and swelling in the joints in addition to significant stiffness and pain.

It is believed that the inflammation of RA causes other problems, too. People with RA often have such symptoms as fatigue, low-grade fever, decreased appetite, depression, and muscle aches, along with pain and swelling in their joints. In fact, many people with RA say that they just don't feel well. These people are describing **malaise,** a vague feeling of illness. This overall feeling of illness is common with RA because the condition is **systemic,** meaning that it can affect more than one part of the body. RA is also referred to as a **chronic** illness because it can last for months or years.

Which joints are involved in RA varies from one person to another. For example, some people have painful joints only in their hands, whereas others may experience pain in their knees or feet. One of the distinguishing characteristics of RA, however, is the particular pattern of specific joints that can potentially become affected. Those most commonly involved in RA are finger joints, wrists, elbows, shoulders, some joints in the neck, jaw, hips, knees, ankles, and foot and toe joints (see Figure 1). RA most often affects the body symmetrically, meaning that arthritis on one side of the body matches that on the other.

One condition that is often confused with RA by patients and physicians is **osteoarthritis** (OA), also called *degenerative joint disease* (DJD). OA is quite different from RA. For one thing, OA is much more common than RA, affecting about sixteen million people in the United States alone.

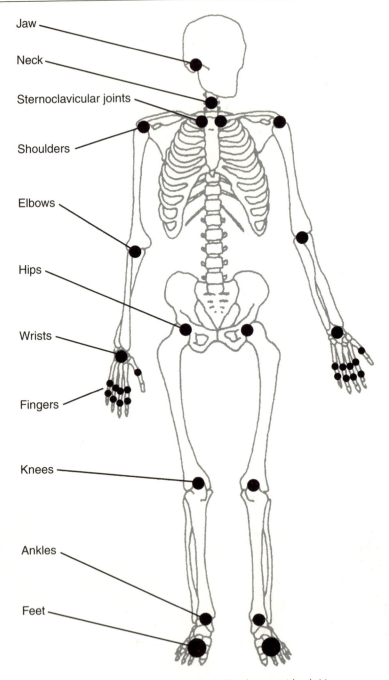

Jaw

Neck

Sternoclavicular joints

Shoulders

Elbows

Hips

Wrists

Fingers

Knees

Ankles

Feet

Figure 1. Joints commonly affected by rheumatoid arthritis

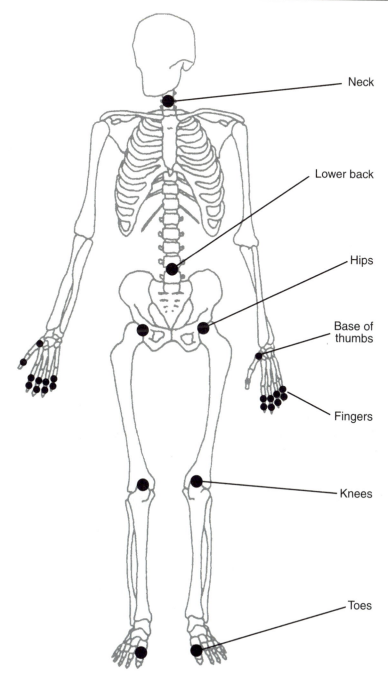

Neck

Lower back

Hips

Base of
thumbs

Fingers

Knees

Toes

Figure 2. Joints commonly affected by osteoarthritis

In fact, nearly all of us will develop OA to some degree as we get older. The distribution pattern of joints affected by OA is different from that of RA, but as you can see by comparing Figures 1 and 2, some joints can be affected in both conditions. This is one of the causes of diagnostic confusion between these two forms of arthritis. Furthermore, some people have both OA and RA.

What causes RA? Researchers, physicians, epidemiologists, theologians, and complementary practitioners have devoted an enormous amount of time and energy to trying to answer this question. Despite their efforts over the past century (since the question was first posed, by Sir Archibald Garrod, in 1858 when he named rheumatoid arthritis), no single cause of RA has been identified.

We have understood for some time that genetics plays a role in the development of RA. We also know that genes alone do not tell the whole story. The tendency for RA to run in families is not high. For patients with RA, the risks for siblings to develop the condition is 2 to 3 percent. Hence, we know that RA is not inherited in the usual sense—that is, passed directly from parent to child. Genes creating susceptibility are inherited, however. Because of our recent success in mapping the human genome, we are much closer to understanding which specific genes contribute to the risk of developing RA. A major family study is under way in Europe and in the United States. The National Institutes of Health and the Arthritis Foundation have joined forces to form the North American Rheumatoid Arthritis Consortium. This group of researchers is collecting medical information and genetic information from families with two or more siblings with RA. This study will be looking at more than 1,000 sibling pairs with RA, to determine common genes they may possess. This will be a national resource for genetic studies. This and other studies will certainly give us specific details on genetic markers that can be present in people with RA. Several years ago genetic markers, HLA-DR4 and DR1, were identified in some people with RA. Many experts believe that there are several other genes involved. Researchers in Iceland recently mapped another gene found in families predisposed to RA. Genetic markers may some day help us direct treatment for RA.

We already know that not everyone with genetic markers for RA develops the condition. It has long been suspected that a virus, a bacterium, or another unknown microbe triggers the development of RA in people made susceptible by their genetic makeup. In 1912, Frank Billings proposed that RA was a response to chronic infection. Over the past century, scientists have searched for a link between hundreds of different infections and the development of RA. In the late 1920s tuberculosis was the suspected culprit. Other bacterial suspects have included streptococci, *Mycoplasma,* and intestinal bacteria such as *E. coli* and *Proteus.* More recently, we have focused on viruses, such as Epstein-Barr virus, Rubella, and Parvovirus. Despite hundreds of theories involving different microbes, and some fascinating discoveries, a clear trigger for RA has not been proven.

People are often concerned about whether someone can "catch" RA from another person. In 1950, two investigators *tried* to transmit RA to volunteers, by injecting into their joints fluid taken from the joints of people with RA (Levinski and Lansbury 1951). Thankfully, no volunteers developed RA. This was early evidence that RA did not appear to be a persistent *infection* of the joints. Currently, scientists are using sophisticated techniques to make certain that there are no signs of microbes in an affected joint. Whether or not evidence of previous infection is found, we are quite convinced that *RA is not contagious.*

We are getting closer to delineating the genetic prerequisites for RA. New techniques will, we hope, help us identify presumed infectious triggers or the "footprints" of these microbes. Research will then be directed at determining how environmental and genetic factors interact to cause and perpetuate the symptoms and effects of RA. We will likely discover that there are several different conditions included in what we now call rheumatoid arthritis. Unraveling the complex series of events that causes RA will give us new and exciting opportunities to treat and one day cure RA.

For More Information

Arthritis Foundation, 1330 West Peachtree St., Atlanta, Ga. 30309; e-mail: help@arthritis.org; Web site: www.arthritis.org; toll-free telephone numbers: 1-800-283-7800 (automated information and to request brochures), 1-800-207-8633 (to order books), 1-404-872-7100 (general questions), 1-800-933-0032 (membership information)

National Institute of Arthritis and Musculoskeletal and Skin Diseases (NIAMS), Information Clearinghouse, NIAMS/National Institutes of Health, 1 AMS Circle, Bethesda, Md. 20892-3675; Web sites: www.nih.gov/niams; (to order NIH/NIAMS–sponsored pamphlet on RA): Consumer Information Center at www.pueblo.gsa.gov/cic_text/health/rheumatoid/rheumatoid.txt; toll-free telephone number: 1-877-226-4267

PART I

Learning about Rheumatoid Arthritis

·

CHAPTER 1

The Joints and Rheumatoid Arthritis

•

The human body has more than one hundred joints. In the adult body many of these joints move very little or not at all, and we are mostly unaware of them. In this chapter we will describe the anatomy and function of the joints, before turning to a discussion of the joint in rheumatoid arthritis (RA).

The Joints

The joints may be divided into three basic types according to the amount of motion each permits: rigid, slightly mobile, and freely movable. The different types of joints work in different ways to achieve different functions.

Rigid Joints

The joints that separate the bones in the skull and pelvis are examples of rigid, or fixed, joints. These joints are movable only during infancy, to allow for growth, or in special circumstances, such as pregnancy, to accommodate delivery. These joints are not affected by RA.

Slightly Mobile Joints

Some joints, such as those between the vertebrae in the spine, normally move only slightly. The vertebrae (bones) are separated by a cushion of **cartilage** called a *disk*. In fact, when these joints move more than a very little bit, problems can arise. A "slipped disk," for example, occurs when the slightly mobile disk moves farther than it should. These joints are not affected in RA.

Freely Movable Joints

Freely movable joints, known as *synovial joints* or *disarthrodial joints,* are the kinds of joints most people think of when asked to name a joint. The shoulders, elbows, wrists, finger and toe joints, hips, knees, and ankles are all freely movable joints. Synovial joints can be affected by RA.

There are great differences among the various synovial joints in terms of structure and function. For instance, the knee and elbow joints permit motion primarily in one direction, because the contours of the bones on either side of these joints fit together like a hinge. The hip and shoulder joints, however, allow movement in many directions. To accommodate this wide range of motion, these joints are built like a ball and socket.

Although different synovial joints function in different ways, all of them are composed of the same parts.

What Are the Parts of a Synovial Joint?

Synovial joints are composed of supportive structures, including the cartilage, tendon, ligament, and muscle, made up of various kinds of **tissue.** Each type of tissue, in turn, is made up of specialized **cells,** which give it one or more specific properties that allow the joint to function normally. The properties of the tissue in the different structures which contribute to proper joint function include resilience, elasticity, compressibility, and strength. (The major parts of a synovial joint are illustrated in Figure 3.)

The *joint capsule* is a fibrous wrapping that encloses the structures within the true joint. (Fibrous tissue is made up of slender, threadlike structures.) This resilient tissue is similar to the "gristle" in a tough steak.

The synovial membrane, or *synovium,* is the lining inside the joint capsule. This smooth, thin membrane is normally composed of a fine layer of cells. It has a rich blood supply that allows nutrients to be delivered to the inside of the joints. The synovium and its cells produce a liquid called *synovial fluid* (or *joint fluid*), which both lubricates and helps nourish the joints. One component of this fluid is a lubricating substance called *hyaluronic acid,* which is secreted by the synovial lining cells. In the normal joint, a small amount of this fluid keeps the cartilage surface lubricated and reduces friction during movement of the joint.

Cartilage is the covering for the ends of the bone. This tissue is made up of cells called chondrocytes, which are embedded in the surrounding material called *cartilage matrix.* Cartilage has a slippery surface that compresses easily and glides smoothly when the joint moves. The spongelike compressibility of cartilage allows it to soak up fluid and nutrients produced by the synovial membrane. A strong framework of connective tissue fibers called **collagen** holds the cartilage together and gives it durabil-

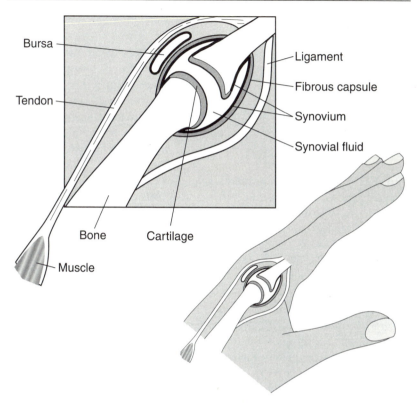

Figure 3. Normal synovial joint

ity. The sophisticated design of cartilage allows it to compress during impact while retaining its glossy surface to minimize friction. This provides a cushion for the bones. Unlike the synovial membrane, the cartilage has no direct blood supply; this may limit its ability to heal when injured.

Bone is found on both sides of a joint. Like cartilage, bone has living cells within its substance. Strong and durable, bone makes a suitable material for our body framework. Because of its rigidity, however, bone can fracture under mechanical stress. The area of bone directly under the cartilage, known as the subchondral bone, is often damaged in RA.

Ligaments are the cordlike structures that attach one bone to another bone across a joint. These cords are much like sturdy guy wires, and they stabilize the joints so that the joints bend only in the direction in which they were intended to bend. For instance, the knee can either bend (**flexion**) or straighten out (**extension**). Ligaments on the sides of the knee prevent the joint from moving to either side when the knee is flexing. Other ligaments stop the knee from bending back on itself when the leg is fully extended.

Muscles are important contributors to joint function and stability. They serve as stabilizers and protectors of joints in addition to being the source of power for all movement. As you might expect, muscles provide the strength required to allow movement to take place at the joint. Combinations of muscles acting in unison can result in a wide range of motions. This is how we can use the same joint (the shoulder) to reach behind our back, across our chest, and over our head. We do so by activating different muscle groups.

In addition to movement, the muscles also provide stability for a joint in a given position. For instance, if you raise your arms to comb your hair, certain muscle groups contract to lift your arms above your head. After your arms are raised, the muscles continue to work to keep your arms elevated while you use your hands and wrists to comb your hair. Similarly, when you are standing in line without moving, your muscles remain contracted, to allow your body to stand erect without collapsing at the hips or knees. Even without movement, then, muscles are critical: they allow us to retain the stationary position of our joints.

Lastly, muscles automatically protect the joints during movement, without requiring conscious thought on our part. As an illustration of this property of muscles, recall the last time you unexpectedly missed a step while walking down a set of stairs. Your muscles did not expect or prepare for the missed step, and your knee or hip felt the jolt of unprotected movement. If the step had been anticipated, the appropriate muscles would have contracted, acting much like a shock absorber on a car, to protect the joints for the step. This automatic protection function of the muscles results in a reduction of the impact on the joints in the course of daily living.

Muscles are attached to bone by *tendons*, which are similar to ligaments except that they connect muscle to bone instead of bone to bone. Because the tendons are located at the end of muscles, they move when muscles tighten, or contract. To demonstrate this to yourself, bend your arm at your elbow. At the same time, feel the area on the inside of your elbow for a ropelike structure at the end of the biceps muscle. This is a tendon.

The tendon is surrounded by an envelope known as the *tendon sheath,* in which the tendon slides back and forth. This sheath has a lining (similar to the synovial membrane) which permits easy gliding. When muscle tendons are in good health, they provide excellent support for the joint, much as ligaments do. Tendons and their tendon sheath can become inflamed, however, from overuse (producing a condition called *tendinitis*) or from RA (producing a condition called **tenosynovitis**).

Another structure located near the joints which helps the tendons and muscles move smoothly over bone is the **bursa**. Bursae are sacs, located between or under muscles, which help the muscles slide without resistance or friction. If these structures become inflamed they can become filled with fluid, a condition known as **bursitis**.

The Joints in RA

When considering how RA affects the joints and why it produces some of the symptoms it does, it is important to recognize that no two people with RA are exactly alike. The severity of RA varies from person to person and joint to joint. Because of these differences it is often difficult to assess precisely how much joint damage is present.

What Is Inflammation?

Our body has a natural defense mechanism to fight off illness and disease. It is called the immune system. *Inflammation* is a common but complicated process that our bodies experience as a response to injury or infection. Inflammation is actually part of the body's immune system response to the injury or infection. Whenever we cut or burn ourselves, for example, inflammation occurs. Inflammation also occurs at the site of an infection (a person with bronchitis, for example, has inflamed bronchi, or airways). The symptoms and signs of inflammation are warmth, pain, redness, and swelling. The amount of inflammation involved is usually proportional to the severity of the injury or infection.

Under normal circumstances, unique **white blood cells** called **lymphocytes, neutrophils,** and **macrophages** strategically interact with one another to accomplish controlled inflammation. When the goal is fighting an infection, this team of cells work together to defend the body from the foreign invader causing the infection. They communicate with each other by chemical messengers called *cytokines*. In the process of fighting infection, cells produce noxious substances which cause the symptoms of inflammation. Again, under normal circumstances, after the infection is cleared, the cells retreat, and inflammation subsides. In these situations inflammatory cells are extremely useful in protecting the body. After an injury, the goal of these white blood cells is healing, and they work together to accomplish this goal.

Inflammation is usually self-limiting in that it goes away by itself after the infection is cleared from the body. As the infection goes away or the wound is healed and repaired, the signs of inflammation resolve as well.

How Is the Inflammation of RA Different
from Normal Inflammation?

The inflammation that occurs in RA involves the white cells mentioned above, but the inciting event—the cause—of the inflammation, is unknown. This trigger could be a virus or another foreign substance or **antigen** (something that is foreign to the body). Normally, antigens are removed and destroyed by the body's immune system. Some theories hold that it is this process that has gone awry in RA.

When a protective cell called the macrophage hooks up to the antigen (or foreign invader), it stimulates an increase in the number of lymphocytes. Two types of lymphocytes, T and B cells, generally play an integral but self-limited role in fighting infection. In RA these cells become chronically "overexcited," and this overexcited state works to maintain inflammation in the joints. Continued inflammation produces the heat, swelling, and pain of arthritis—and damage to joints.

In RA, the body launches a continuous immune response. When no known antigen is present, the body appears to fight against itself. Therefore, RA is often called an *autoimmune disease*. Immune cells mistakenly react against the body, causing inflammation.

The Stages of RA: How Does Inflammation Affect the Joints?

RA may be divided into five stages. Each stage is characterized by the status of the *uncontrolled* inflammation present in the joints.

Stage 1 (normal). In this stage, people with RA have no symptoms of arthritis, and their joints appear normal (Figure 3). Some of these people may be genetically susceptible to arthritis (see the Introduction). Having an RA gene marker alone is not sufficient to cause someone to develop RA, however. It is presumed that some unknown trigger initiates the development of arthritis in the genetically susceptible person; that is, an unknown factor triggers the inflammatory process, and other unknown factors keep it going, apparently blocking normal resolution of the inflammation. One theory is that in RA, the communication between cells is disturbed in some way, allowing ongoing inflammation to occur.

Stage 2. This is the stage during which people with RA first have symptoms. Early in the course of arthritis, small lymphocytes migrate to the synovial lining, causing what is called **synovitis,** or inflammation of the synovium (see Figure 4). The macrophages and lymphocytes continue to promote inflammation by producing cytokines, "chemical messengers" that are responsible for delivering messages from one part of the body to

Synovitis

Figure 4. Stage 2 rheumatoid arthritis

another. Two specific cytokines, *tumor necrosis factor* (*TNF*) and *interleukin-1* (*IL-1*) have been identified as significantly increasing inflammation. People with RA have increased amounts of TNF and IL-1 in their joints. Cytokines can induce an increase in the number of blood vessels going to the synovium, and with increased blood flow, the joints become warm. The leakage of cytokines into the bloodstream may also contribute to the fatigue that is so common in RA. Other cytokines are partially responsible for stimulating cells to produce prostaglandins and leukotrienes, both of which are potent producers of inflammation. Continued production of cytokines, prostaglandins, leukotrienes, and other substances leads to swelling, warmth, and pain in the joints. In Chapter 14 we describe how this knowledge about cytokines translates into effective treatment options for controlling symptoms of RA.

It is also during stage 2 that B lymphocytes are transformed into another type of white blood cell, the **plasma cell,** which manufactures **antibodies.** Antibodies, also referred to as *immunoglobulins*, are distinctive proteins that the body normally produces to fight against viruses and foreign bacteria, ones not normally present in the body. In RA, for reasons that are unclear, the body appears to produce an excessive amount of antibodies. One particular antibody often found in the blood of people with RA is called the **rheumatoid factor.** The production of rheumatoid factor exacerbates the inflammatory process. (Rheumatoid factors are discussed in more detail in Chapter 3.)

Stage 3. In this stage there is a marked increase in the number of cells in the synovium, possibly stimulated by the presence of various cytokines. The synovium becomes much thicker, or **hypertrophied,** and this makes the joint feel doughy or spongy (see Figure 5). An increase in the amount of synovial fluid in the joint adds to the stiffness and limitation of motion of the joints. (Accumulation of joint fluid is known as *joint effusion.*)

With RA there is also an increase in hyaluronic acid, the lubricating substance in the synovial joint fluid. Many people believe that increased hyaluronic acid is responsible for morning stiffness (or morning **gelling**) and the stiffness experienced after sitting for a prolonged period of time without moving (gelling phenomenon).

Joint fluid contains inflammatory white blood cells called neutrophils (or polymorphonuclear leukocytes). (Why lymphocytes reside in the synovial lining and neutrophils appear in the synovial fluid is unclear.) In the joint affected by RA, neutrophils join lymphocytes in perpetuating the inflammatory process. In testing for RA, the physician may remove a sample of fluid from the joints to determine the relative proportions of these cells present. This helps the physician differentiate RA from other forms of arthritis.

A person in any one of the three earliest stages of RA may experience significant joint symptoms, including pain, heat, swelling, stiffness, and loss of motion. All of these inflammatory changes are potentially reversible with proper medical therapy.

Synovial
hypertrophy

Joint
effusion

Figure 5. Stage 3 rheumatoid arthritis

Stage 4. At this point, inflamed synovium can grow (proliferate), spreading over the top of joint cartilage (Figure 6). When synovium grows in this way, it is called *pannus*. The pannus produces enzymes called *collagenases,* which can destroy collagen, the cartilage proteins. Neutrophils in the joint fluid can also release harmful enzymes. Although there are many beneficial enzymes in the body, these particular enzymes can break down, or degrade, the cartilage that protects the bone and joints.

Collagenases can also cause bone to break down in the area in which the synovitis meets bone. This results in the formation of tiny holes or **erosions** in the bone and cartilage. Erosions often occur first at the point at which protective cartilage ends at the margins of joints.

Stage 5. If the arthritis is left untreated, the pannus can further invade and erode through cartilage and bone by producing more enzymes. Any loss of cartilage reduces the amount of cushioning between the bones of the joint (Figure 7).

When cartilage is roughened by this erosion, the ability to have smooth joint motion is lost. People with RA can feel a grating sensation in the joint during movement, and their physicians can feel the grating of the joint during physical examination. This grating is called *crepitus.* If the breakdown of cartilage is persistent, the cartilage can be totally eroded by pannus.

In stage 5 RA, uncontrolled swelling can cause ligaments and tendons to stretch, adding to the *instability* of the joint. Muscles become smaller

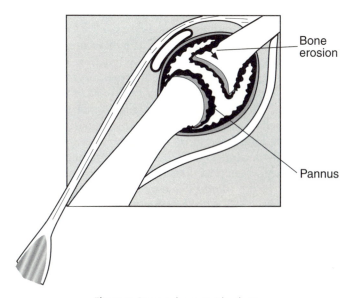

Figure 6. Stage 4 rheumatoid arthritis

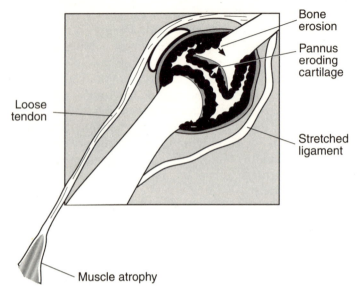

Bone
erosion

Pannus
eroding
cartilage

Loose
tendon

Stretched
ligament

Muscle atrophy

Figure 7. Stage 5 rheumatoid arthritis

(**atrophy**) and weaker because of disuse. Stretched ligaments and tendons and atrophied muscles interfere with the joint's ability to function properly, often resulting in a joint that does not move as it was intended to. Inflammation and pannus can spread along the tendons in tenosynovitis, making the tendons weak and putting them at risk for rupture. When the cartilage is eroded and the supporting structures are loosened, other changes often occur which alter the shape and function of the joint. These mechanical changes are a result more of abnormal forces occurring across the joint than of ongoing inflammation in the joint itself.

Late in this stage, after the cartilage is totally eroded, the amount of inflammation and swelling often decreases, producing what is sometimes referred to as a *burned-out joint*. At this stage the stretched ligaments and tendons can actually become even looser, as the swelling pushing against them decreases. The looseness of these supporting structures can seriously affect the stability of the joint. (These changes and the prevention and treatment of them are discussed throughout this book.)

Summary

Of the three major types of joints in the body, only synovial joints are affected by RA. All the parts of the joint play a role in normal function:

· The *capsule* encloses and protects the joint.
· The *synovium* provides lubrication and nutrition for the joint.
· *Cartilage* cushions and reduces friction with movement.
· *Bone* provides structure.
· *Ligaments* and *tendons* support the joint.
· *Muscles* provide joint movement, protection, and stability.
· *Bursae* decrease friction with movement.

Early symptoms of RA include pain, swelling, warmth, and stiffness (especially in the morning) in the joints, and mild restriction of motion. Joint symptoms and such generalized symptoms as fatigue are caused by a variety of inflammatory substances which are produced by different cells.

In RA, for unknown reasons, the normal cells of the joint lining and white blood cells become overactivated, resulting in uncontrolled inflammation in the joints.

Early stages of RA are often reversible with timely medical therapy.

CHAPTER 2

The Course and Prognosis of Rheumatoid Arthritis

•

For most people with rheumatoid arthritis (RA), questions about the future course of their condition are of major concern. Anyone who has been diagnosed with RA will naturally want and need answers to these questions to make plans for the future. Physicians and other health professionals will answer these questions as best as they can given the present state of knowledge about the course of RA and what they know about an individual's specific condition.

Like many other chronic illnesses, however, RA is often unpredictable. The onset of RA may be gradual or sudden, with one or many joints affected. The course of arthritis is also varied, and it may even change over time in the same person. For these reasons it is important to keep in mind that any prediction made by health care professionals about the future course of RA in any one individual is a guess—an educated guess, but a guess.

The questions people with RA most commonly ask about the future are presented in this chapter along with the best answers the medical professional can provide at this time.

The Course of RA

How Does RA Usually Start?

Variability is the key ingredient in the answer to this question. Most commonly, RA starts gradually, with pain and stiffness in one or more of the joints noted in Figure 1. Usually, people first notice these symptoms in their hands. Early on, swelling may not be apparent, despite sensations of pain or stiffness. As the amount of pain slowly increases, however, swelling becomes obvious. Swelling in the joints usually appears within months of the onset of pain in the joints. Rarely, swelling does not appear until years after pain begins.

For seven out of ten people with RA, the symptoms of arthritis appear in matching joints, on both sides of the body; this is called *symmetrical arthritis*. For example, the left and right wrists may both be affected or the left and right knees. In addition to feeling pain in the joints, people experiencing the early symptoms of RA may feel very fatigued, as though they were recovering from a cold or the flu.

For some people, RA begins differently. These people may notice only increasing stiffness (particularly in the morning) without experiencing a great deal of pain. Others notice only progressively severe swelling, initially without pain. Still other people experience bouts of joint pain or swelling which appear suddenly and then disappear just as quickly. Someone who has these recurring attacks or flare-ups of arthritis which resolve quickly may be given a diagnosis of *palindromic rheumatism* before diagnostic evidence for RA develops.

Less commonly, RA can begin with only one or two tender, swollen joints in an asymmetrical pattern, that is, the joints affected on one side of the body are different from the joints affected on the other side of the body. Since this is an unusual way for RA to begin, health care providers may be hesitant about confirming a diagnosis of RA based on these symptoms. In time, about half of the people whose joint pain begins in an asymmetrical pattern will develop the more typical symmetrical pattern of RA.

RA sometimes begins as aching and stiff muscles, particularly in the shoulders and hips. This nonspecific aching may continue for weeks or months before the swelling of joints appears. Older individuals are more likely than younger people to have muscle aches and stiffness appear as the first sign of RA.

Finally, RA may appear as rapid onset arthritis, with swelling and pain in many joints as well as such systemic symptoms as severe fatigue, low-grade fever, loss of appetite, and weight loss seemingly developing overnight.

What Course of Arthritis Can I Expect?

After you have been diagnosed with RA you will wonder what course or *natural history* your arthritis will follow. Will it continue in the same way it started, or will additional, or different, joints become involved in time? The answers to these questions are as different as the persons asking them. In some cases, the way arthritis starts allows physicians to predict the course it will follow, but this is not true in every case.

The following four general courses that RA can follow were described *before* current treatments (or therapeutic strategies) had been developed, and therefore they reflect the natural histories *untreated* of RA (Figure 8). Keep in mind that what follows are four *potential* courses of *untreated* RA. The actual course of any given individual's RA may vary from any of these four courses.

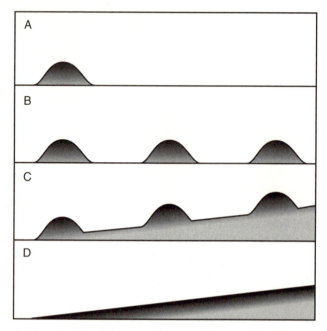

Figure 8. Potential courses of untreated rheumatoid arthritis

1. Spontaneous remission (Figure 8A). The person who develops signs and symptoms of RA and then, with little or no medication (generally only *nonsteroidal anti-inflammatory medications,* **NSAIDs**), becomes symptom-free, is said to have gone into spontaneous remission. Remission may be described as a period of time during which there is no evidence of active disease or illness, in this case, RA.

During remission from RA, blood tests, such as the **erythrocyte sedimentation rate** *(ESR)* or C reactive protein (**CRP**) (see Chapter 3), often produce normal results. Generally it is estimated that 20 percent of all RA patients will have a spontaneous remission, but more than 50 percent of these will have a recurrence of RA in the future. Thus, in reality, probably only 5 to 10 percent of untreated patients have a permanent remission. The majority of people with RA require continued treatment.

Patients and physicians often wonder how long they should wait for this potential spontaneous remission before starting stronger medications designed to bring on a medically induced remission (these medications are called **DMARDs,** or disease-modifying antirheumatic drugs). The optimal time to start DMARDs varies from case to case, but most rheumatologists would begin if there was any evidence of impending joint damage and certainly if joint damage was visible on x-ray films. This is particularly important since it is now generally believed that these drugs are most effective if taken early in the course of arthritis.

2. Remitting (Figure 8B). Some people with RA have a series of flare-ups of arthritis followed by a return to normal health between attacks. A person who has remitting arthritis may not need remission-inducing medications if there is no ongoing joint damage and if joint function returns to normal between flare-ups. The attacks themselves, when the arthritis is active, are commonly treated with NSAIDs. Attacks that occur very frequently or that are very lengthy may begin to affect the person's life-style, and then the person with RA and the physician may decide that DMARDs should be taken.

3. Remitting progressive (Figure 8C). The third possible course of RA is one in which the person experiences a pattern of flare-ups without a return to normal health between attacks. Joint damage over time is a distinct possibility in this course of RA, because some inflammation remains in the joints between attacks. In this case, DMARD therapy ought to be a serious consideration.

4. Progressive (Figure 8D). In this course, the person experiences a gradual increase in pain, swelling, and joint damage over time. Usually this progression occurs very slowly, but some people experience a rapid loss of function. Early treatment with DMARD therapy in an effort to halt progression of arthritis is recommended.

Can a Remission Be Brought on with Medications?

As stated above, DMARDs, and now a new group of medications called biologic response modifiers (BRMs), are used in an attempt to induce a remission of RA, and many people achieve improvement by taking one of these medications. (For more information about NSAIDs, DMARDs, and BRMs, see Chapters 12, 13, and 14.) Unfortunately, it is not always possible to predict which of the many medications will bring about improvement for a specific individual. One drug may induce a remission in one person and not work very well for the next. For this reason, prescribing the proper medication often involves a trial-and-error approach coupled with close communication between the patient and the physician.

Different medications have different potential side effects, all of which your doctor will discuss with you. (These are described in detail in Part IV.) It is very important to keep in mind that *no two people are alike in the way they respond to medications;* this means, among other things, that the risk for medication side effects and allergies varies from one person to the next. Therefore, when decisions are being made about which medication is best suited to you, *thoughtful, ongoing communication between you and your physician is essential.*

There are two principles that hold true for drugs that are intended to induce a remission. One is that early treatment is probably most effective. You must decide for yourself whether the potential benefits of early treatment, aimed at preventing permanent joint damage, outweigh possible medication toxicities. With your physician's guidance, you must balance risks, make informed decisions, and set realistic goals.

The second principle is that by their nature, DMARDs work slowly. In most cases inflammation did not develop instantaneously, and it is unlikely to resolve rapidly, even with appropriate therapy. Most medications aimed at remission take several weeks or months to work. For this reason, patience is required; you need to reserve judgment about the effectiveness of a medication until an adequate trial treatment has elapsed. Improvement with a DMARD may take weeks to months. The newest class of disease-modifying drugs, the biologic response modifiers, appears to have a faster response time than the older DMARDs. People will often see results in weeks rather than months. (See Chapter 14.)

As discussed in Chapter 12, NSAIDs are a group of medications aimed at reducing inflammation. NSAIDs are effective drugs that often reduce pain and inflammation quickly (days to weeks) compared with DMARDs. Nevertheless, however helpful they may be in controlling symptoms, NSAIDs probably have little effect on the course of RA.

We remain very optimistic about the effectiveness of our present medications and can assure you that many new medications are currently under intensive investigation. It is important to avoid becoming discouraged if one medicine fails, because very possibly the next medication you try will work for you. Also, there are various methods for controlling pain, preventing joint damage, and improving function while waiting for the medications to take effect (these methods are discussed later in this book).

The Prognosis of RA

Can Arthritis Be Cured?

RA is generally a **chronic** condition in which true cures or permanent remissions are unusual with the medications presently available. This does not mean that most cases of arthritis cannot be controlled effectively, however. The majority of people with RA achieve good to excellent control with a treatment program consisting of medications, therapeutic exercise, adequate rest, and proper joint protection. And most people with

RA are able to continue with their normal activities, with some minor adjustments to accommodate joint changes that have occurred.

Will Other Joints Become Involved with Time?

Possibly. Most people initially develop pain in their hands and wrists, and it is likely that they will experience at the least some discomfort in other joints. But not all joints are affected equally by RA in all people. For instance, the person who is having significant pain and difficulties with finger joints will not necessarily experience the same degree of inflammation or pain in any other joints.

Will I Become Disabled?

Today, treatment of RA begins earlier in the course of the condition, and treatment options are more varied and more effective. The currently available medications can be very effective, and many more are under intensive investigation. Today, too, there is an appreciation of the value of therapeutic exercise, and new methods have been developed to protect joints in order to avoid disability. Even in the least successful cases, in which arthritis persists despite the medical team's efforts, other options remain. Also, the many surgical procedures available today are infinitely more effective than those offered a few decades ago.

Will you become disabled? Today, the odds against this are overwhelmingly in your favor, which is why it is best to avoid listening to a well-meaning friend's stories about her great-aunt who lives a wheelchairbound life because of RA. Remember, each person's case is different, and so much has changed in the approach to treating RA that comparisons are just not valid. The fact that you are reading a book about your condition and taking an active role in making decisions about treatment proves that you are different from the patients of a half-century ago.

Will you need to make some life-style changes? Yes, but that in no way means that you need to relinquish any of your life goals. If you have a good understanding of how to control the particular problems associated with your arthritis and if you remain open to learning new ways to make adjustments, you will succeed in living a normal, productive life. Will you be inconvenienced? Yes, definitely. Will you be disabled? Highly unlikely.

Does RA Shorten a Person's Life?

RA, like most chronic illnesses, is associated with a very slight decrease in life span when all patients who have RA are compared with people who are free of illness. This may not have any individual significance for you, because these statistics are derived from comparisons of large groups of people. Therefore, if you are otherwise healthy, you have an excellent chance of living a full and long life.

A very small minority of people with severe RA (less than 5 percent) develop complications that make them very ill. These individuals have life-threatening conditions (discussed in Chapter 4).

Summary

Rheumatoid arthritis begins in different ways and can follow a wide variety of potential courses.

RA responds best when treated early.

DMARDs, or disease-modifying antirheumatic drugs, can bring about an improvement in many people.

NSAIDs, or nonsteroidal anti-inflammatory drugs, can quickly ease the symptoms of inflammation and pain, but they are less effective than DMARDs in changing the course of RA.

BRMs, or biologic response modifiers, are the latest class of disease-modifying drugs and work more quickly than traditional DMARDs.

Although true cures are unlikely, excellent control of arthritis is possible with a comprehensive treatment program.

Most people with RA live normal, full lives with some minor life-style adjustments.

CHAPTER 3

Diagnosing Rheumatoid Arthritis: Why So Many Tests?

•

You may be wondering why it took so long or was so difficult for your doctor to diagnose your rheumatoid arthritis (RA). It may have appeared at first that the physician was hedging on the diagnosis or refusing to provide you with a diagnosis on the spot. Because there are so many different ailments that can cause pain in the joints and so many different kinds of arthritis, the physician needed time to determine which was affecting you. And, as discussed in Chapter 2, the pain of RA begins a little differently in each person; that is to say, there is no one set of symptoms by which the doctor can identify RA immediately.

It may be helpful to review the initial steps taken in reaching a diagnosis of RA: the clinical history, the physical examination, and a **differential diagnosis.** Early in the course of RA, diagnostic tests (for example, blood tests and x-rays) may not be able to confirm a diagnosis of RA, although they can sometimes rule out other conditions whose symptoms resemble those of RA. Diagnostic tests can *help* identify RA in later stages.

Clinical History

The most valuable information you can provide to your doctor on an initial visit is your clinical history. Usually the doctor will ask you to describe your symptoms and then will ask you specific questions about your symptoms, such as:

· Which joints are painful or stiff?
· When is the pain or stiffness worse?
· What makes the symptoms better or worse?
· How long does the morning stiffness last?
· Do you feel tired much of the time?

Providing your physician with complete and accurate answers to these questions is one of the most important roles you can play in your own medical care. This is because the physician depends on an analysis of the clinical history to help identify the cause of your joint problems.

It's a good idea to prepare a written record of your symptoms as they occur. You can draw up a list of symptoms, including where you feel pain or stiffness or swelling and the time of day when it occurs or when it is the most bothersome; take this list with you to the doctor's office. This list will help you answer your doctor's questions accurately because you will have a written record of what you have been experiencing before your visit. Not everyone can remember *exactly* when pain or stiffness or swelling was *first* experienced or pinpoint the onset of changes in ability to perform a given task. Once you become aware of these changes, however, it is a good idea to keep a record of them.

Physical Examination

After the clinical history is taken, the physician will perform a physical examination. Your physician will examine all of your joints, looking for evidence of tenderness, heat, swelling, and decreased motion. Your doctor will pay particular attention to the pattern of joint involvement, because one of the distinguishing characteristics of RA is the particular pattern of joints that can be affected. Often the physician will perform a *complete* physical examination (including taking your blood pressure; feeling your glands; examining your eyes, ears, nose, throat, and skin; listening to your heart and lungs; examining your abdomen; and checking your reflexes and muscle strength) to uncover clues to help him or her identify the type of arthritis you have.

Sometimes, in the early stages of RA, people find the results of the physical examination frustrating, because they are experiencing significant pain or stiffness in their joints and the physician may not be able to detect outward signs of joint inflammation. In these cases the physician has to proceed on the basis of the patient's description of the pain or stiffness he or she is experiencing. Again, the accuracy of the clinical history provided to the physician is extremely important.

Differential Diagnosis

After the physical examination, the physician will develop a differential diagnosis. This consists of a list of possible causes of your specific symptoms. The physician will order specific laboratory tests to rule out certain of the diagnoses and other tests to confirm the proper diagnosis (these tests are described in detail below).

As we will see, blood tests and x-rays are seldom helpful in diagnosing RA in the very earliest stage. For this reason, your tests may not uncover any specific abnormalities. On the one hand, you'll probably be happy that the test results are normal; on the other hand, there's the frustration of knowing that something is wrong and not having a test result to prove it. Your physician may temporarily have to make an experienced best guess of the diagnosis in this case. Effective treatment can be initiated before test results are diagnostically significant, however.

What Makes RA So Difficult to Diagnose?

RA is the most common of the inflammatory forms of arthritis, and yet making an accurate diagnosis is often difficult. For this reason, your physician may have initially diagnosed your RA as another type of inflammatory arthritis, such as ankylosing spondylitis, Reiter's disease, arthritis associated with psoriasis or colitis, gout, pseudo-gout, or systemic lupus erythematosus (SLE). The symptoms of these forms of arthritis are similar to the symptoms of RA, and many excellent doctors initially misdiagnose RA as being another form of inflammatory arthritis (and vice versa). As mentioned above, RA is also often diagnosed incorrectly as osteoarthritis, the most common form of arthritis.

A good clinical history, a thorough physical examination, some laboratory tests, and a good measure of time and patience are required to diagnose RA. A physician who is well acquainted with the pattern of joint involvement in RA is likely to have an easier time making an accurate diagnosis. Board-certified **rheumatologists** are specifically trained and experienced in making these difficult early diagnoses.

Diagnostic Tests

Physicians rely on diagnostic tests to help them provide quality care to people with RA. Diagnostic tests can take the form of blood analyses, joint fluid analyses, urine analyses, and x-rays. (As might be expected, evaluation of blood and joint fluid requires that a needle be used to obtain specimens.) Diagnostic tests may be requested for any one (or more) of the following reasons:

· To make a diagnosis of RA.
· To monitor disease activity in RA.
· To rule out other types of arthritis.
· To detect complications of RA.
· To screen for potential side effects of a medication.

In addition to laboratory analyses of body fluids and x-ray evaluation, physicians rely heavily on the patient history and physical examination to make a diagnosis of RA, as discussed above. In fact, early in the course of RA, when the results of diagnostic tests may be normal, the physician relies on an evaluation of each person's description of symptoms and the physical exam to make a diagnosis. When the findings from laboratory tests are inconclusive, making the diagnosis often requires a significant amount of observation time. Patience is required from both the physician and the patient in this case.

The following tests may be requested by your physician. As you will see, many of the tests have more than one function. For example, a blood count may be ordered to look for complications of RA or to monitor for side effects of medications.

Most of the tests described below consist of blood or urine analyses, which can be performed in a diagnostic laboratory or in the doctor's office, usually by the doctor's nurse or assistant. Some of the tests, however, are more complicated, and only the skills of an experienced physician can ensure that they are performed safely and accurately. We will identify these procedures in the following section.

What Tests Are Used to Diagnose or Monitor Activity of RA?

Rheumatoid factor, rheumatoid titer. Rheumatoid factor is an antibody found in the blood of 80 to 90 percent of people with RA. A blood test determines whether the antibody is present. The result is often expressed as a *titer,* which is a measurement reflecting the amount of a substance present. The presence of rheumatoid factor *usually* indicates that a diagnosis of RA is accurate, although a change in titer of rheumatoid factor does not necessarily reflect a change in the activity of arthritis.

Erythrocyte sedimentation rate (ESR), or "sed rate." The ESR is a test commonly ordered to monitor inflammation in the body. The test is actually a measurement of how rapidly red blood cells settle (produce sedimentation) in a test tube. When inflammation is present in the body, certain proteins in blood make red blood cells (erythrocytes) settle faster, and this results in a high ESR. It is often useful to monitor the ESR because it can reflect changes in inflammation. A decrease in the ESR suggests that medical treatment has been effective. The ESR is not a very specific test for RA, however, because a high ESR can indicate other conditions, such as infections, that produce significant inflammation.

C reactive protein (CRP). CRP, like ESR, is a test frequently ordered to monitor inflammation level. It sometimes will be elevated when the ESR is not. Many researchers prefer to look at both the ESR and the CRP to get a fuller picture of the degree of inflammation. The CRP should be as low as possible. The therapies that lower it may also limit the damaging effects of RA.

Synovial fluid studies. One of the most helpful tests in rheumatology involves the evaluation of synovial fluid (joint fluid). A **rheumatologist,** an *orthopedic surgeon,* or an experienced primary care physician can remove (aspirate) the fluid from the inflamed or painful joint by needle with minimal discomfort. (The process of puncturing and aspirating a joint is called *arthrocentesis.*) This test is extremely helpful in substantiating a diagnosis of inflammatory arthritis because if the inflammatory white blood cells called **neutrophils** are found to be present in large numbers, and if evidence of other forms of inflammatory arthritis (such as gout crystals) is absent, a diagnosis of RA is supported.

This test is also useful in ruling out other causes of joint swelling or arthritis. Doctors often examine the fluid for the presence of various crystals, which can be seen in the joint fluid of patients with other types of arthritis (gout and pseudo-gout). Different types of crystals cause arthritis, **tendinitis,** and **bursitis.** The crystals that cause gout are composed of uric acid, whereas calcium-containing crystals are responsible for pseudo-gout. It is important to distinguish these conditions from RA because treatment methods for the different conditions vary significantly.

Sampling of the synovial fluid from an inflamed joint is also necessary to evaluate for the presence of infection. This is particularly important when the patient has a fever or is experiencing severe tenderness, swelling, or warmth in a single joint. Even people with established RA may need to be evaluated for infection if one joint is particularly hot and painful.

X-rays. Several types of x-rays are recommended for patients with RA, but the standard x-ray is requested more often than any other kind. Usually hand and foot x-rays are requested, but any symptomatic joint may warrant examination by x-ray. (Remember, it is common for x-rays to be completely normal in the early stages of RA, even for people with severe symptoms.)

The physician will examine the x-rays for signs of such abnormalities as mild thinning of bone (or decreased density) in the areas near the joints (called periarticular demineralization) and, later, the presence of tiny holes in the bones (erosions) and joint space narrowing. As explained in Chapter 1, erosions occur when **synovitis** has damaged **cartilage** and bone. In people with RA the thickness of cartilage can also be reduced by erosion (Figures 6 and 7). When this occurs, the distance between bones (joint space) on x-rays appears smaller than normal. Since only bone can be seen on plain x-rays, and cartilage appears as black space, it is the black space between bones that is measured. Hence, *joint space narrowing* is actually a misnomer, in that the term really means loss of joint cartilage.

X-rays may also be used to rule out other causes of joint pain, including fractures, calcium deposits near the joints, and bone infection.

Standard x-rays of the chest are sometimes taken to rule out a problem in the lungs—a *rare* complication of RA. Some medications for RA (gold, methotrexate, and cyclophosphamide) also cause lung problems—but again, only *rarely*—and x-rays may be taken if symptoms of lung problems develop. Chest x-rays are occasionally scheduled to rule out other highly unusual causes of arthritis which have lung problems associated with them. Standard x-rays can be performed in a physician's office or in a radiology suite.

More sophisticated x-rays, requiring specialized equipment, are used in some situations. These imaging tests include the CAT (computerized axial tomography) scan, or CT scan, the MRI (magnetic resonance imaging), and the bone scan. Unlike standard x-rays, which produce images mostly of bone, CT scans and MRIs also show such tissues as muscle, cartilage, and joint structures. The bone scan is generally performed to seek evidence of inflammation or infection within the bone.

Biopsy. When diagnosis is proving particularly difficult, a biopsy of the **synovium** (*joint lining*) is sometimes required. This procedure involves removing a small piece of the synovium from the joint with a special needle or, more commonly, an arthroscope (an instrument through which the physician can view the inside of the joint). Such a *needle biopsy* is performed in the office by a rheumatologist or an orthopedic surgeon. The skin and tissues are numbed with local anesthetic (usually lidocaine). This procedure usually causes mild discomfort. *Arthroscopic biopsy* is performed in a surgical suite. After a local, spinal, or general anesthetic is administered, a small incision is made. A scope about the diameter of a pencil is then inserted into the joint through the incision. The tissue is generally removed with the same instrument. This procedure usually involves only mild discomfort. The tissue removed allows the doctor to verify the diagnosis of RA and to exclude other conditions.

Biopsy of other tissues in the body, including muscle, nerve, lung, and skin, is indicated in some of the rare complications of RA (discussed in Chapter 4). Successful execution of these biopsy procedures requires the special skills of physicians who have been trained to perform them.

HLA-DR4 and DR-1. In some people these genetic markers are present on the surface of specific white blood cells. Many people with RA—about two-thirds of Caucasians with RA—have these genetic markers, and the presence of these genes *may* indicate that a person is susceptible to developing RA. However, since approximately 25 percent of people who *do not* have RA can have these markers, too, tests for them are not conclusive. Tests for genetic markers are not routinely available and are performed only in research settings or universities.

What Tests Are Used to Rule Out Other Types of Arthritis?

HLA-B27. Blood testing can reveal the presence of another genetic marker, HLA-B27. This marker is often associated with one of several forms of inflammatory arthritis, called *spondylarthropathy,* which can affect the spine as well as tendons and ligaments. Reiter's disease, ankylosing spondylitis, and psoriatic arthritis are all forms of spondylarthropathy. HLA-B27 is also present in about 5 percent of individuals who do not have spondylarthropathy. Therefore, it is not a good diagnostic test.

Antinuclear antibody (ANA), or fluorescent antinuclear antibody (FANA). Testing for this antibody is often requested for people with newly manifested RA symptoms, in an attempt to exclude systemic lupus erythematosus as a diagnosis. Positive (abnormal) results may be an indication of lupus, but a positive result is often obtained in people with RA as well. Other conditions associated with ANA include scleroderma, Sjögren's syndrome, and mixed connective tissue disease. In addition, ANA is present in 5 to 10 percent of people without arthritic problems. This test, then, provides clues but not a definitive answer.

What Tests Are Used to Screen for Complications of RA or Medication Side Effects?

Blood (cell) counts. Three types of blood cells circulate in the bloodstream: red blood cells, white blood cells, and platelets. When all three types of cells are checked through one test, that test is called a *complete blood count* or *CBC.* When specific information is required about the number and percentage of different white blood cell types present, a CBC *with differential* is requested. This test is often used to screen for specific drug side effects and to search for evidence of infection.

Red blood cells help carry oxygen to tissues. When the number of red blood cells decreases, *anemia* results. Anemia can cause a decrease in the delivery of oxygen to tissues because there are fewer red blood cells available to carry oxygen. This decrease in oxygen can result in premature muscle fatigue, decreased stamina, and generalized fatigue and weakness.

Anemia frequently accompanies RA, and it may contribute to the fatigue which many people with RA experience. Anemia is most often a consequence of the **systemic** effects of inflammation on blood, and it often improves as arthritis is treated. However, some medications (nonsteroidal anti-inflammatory drugs, **NSAIDs**) can cause inflammation of the stomach lining and mild blood loss. In this situation, the anemia represents a side effect of medication, which requires further evaluation. The tests used to diagnose and monitor anemia are the **hematocrit** and the **hemoglobin**. Occasionally, a separate test called the reticulocyte count is indicated; this test reflects the rate at which new red blood cells (called *reticulocytes*) are being produced.

The several types of white blood cells include **lymphocytes,** polymorphonuclear leukocytes ("polys" or **neutrophils**), monocytes, basophils, and eosinophils. An important function of white cells is to fight infection; that is, in response to an infection, the body usually produces white blood cells, and a blood test would reveal a higher than normal number of them. Having too few white blood cells may interfere with the body's ability to fight infection. Thus, one side effect of any medication that causes a decrease in the number of white blood cells can be infection.

Platelets perform the clotting function in blood. The platelet count is often either high or low in RA. If the platelet count is too low (*thrombocytopenia*), the risk of excessive or spontaneous bleeding is increased. Some medications lower the platelet count, and again, this requires investigation. High platelet counts (*thrombocytosis*) can occur with chronic inflammation; they generally create no particular problems.

Complement studies. These blood studies, which include tests called C3, C4, and CH50, are used to determine whether a particular part of the immune system is activated. They are rarely performed for people who have an uncomplicated case of RA, but they can be helpful when a person has an unusual complication of RA called *vasculitis* (discussed in Chapter 4).

Liver function tests. Liver function or liver enzyme tests are blood tests that may reflect changes in the liver, such as inflammation and organ damage. Findings of minor abnormalities in these tests are common in RA. Interestingly, though, a change in liver function tests does not necessarily mean that the liver's functioning capacity has been altered. Elevated levels of liver enzymes generally suggest mild liver irritation or past damage. These tests are often used to search for evidence of pre-existing liver problems or to monitor the side effects of medications. Commonly ordered liver function tests include the SGOT (or AST), SGPT (or ALT), LDH, and alkaline phosphatase.

Urinalysis and kidney (renal) function tests. Examination of a urine specimen is an extremely useful test that most often is requested to screen for medication-induced complications affecting the kidneys. Rarely, patients with RA have minor abnormalities in the urine unrelated to medications.

The evaluation of kidney function also requires blood tests called *creatinine* and *blood urea nitrogen* (BUN). The levels of these substances present in the blood indicate how efficiently the kidney is filtering the body's toxins. Sometimes the physician will request a twenty-four-hour urine collection and a blood test, to obtain an extremely accurate assessment of kidney function. Again, these tests are undertaken to monitor for medication side effects or to look for underlying kidney problems.

Bone density testing. Bone density testing is often performed to determine if a person is at risk for **osteoporosis,** a condition which is seen more frequently in patients with RA. (See Chapter 16.) There are several tests that can diagnose this condition. The most informative technique is called the DEXA or Dual-Energy X-Ray Absorptiometry. These tests are noninvasive and readily available. The lower spine and hip region are most commonly measured. The test is very comfortable and does not require needles or medications. It takes approximately 15 minutes to perform. The radiation exposure is very low, markedly less than a normal x-ray. Other techniques include quantitative computed tomography (CT) and quantitative ultrasound.

Summary

The steps taken in reaching a diagnosis of RA are the clinical history, the physical examination, a differential diagnosis, and diagnostic tests.

X-rays and blood tests frequently produce normal results at the onset of arthritis.

Later, an evaluation of blood and joint fluid may be useful in the diagnosis of RA.

Once a diagnosis of RA is made, diagnostic tests may be useful in monitoring a person's condition: blood tests and x-rays can be performed to monitor disease activity and screen for complications of RA, and blood and urine tests are often ordered to screen for medication side effects.

CHAPTER 4

Outside the Joints: Other Symptoms of Rheumatoid Arthritis

•

As a systemic illness, rheumatoid arthritis (RA) can affect more than one part of the body. That is why people with RA often have symptoms that are seemingly unrelated to joint stiffness or swelling. They may be experiencing generalized fatigue, for example, or they may notice a decrease in appetite or run a low-grade fever.

Symptoms or changes occurring outside the joints are called extra-articular features of RA. Some extra-articular features, such as those mentioned above, are very common and cause only minor discomfort or inconvenience; others, such as swollen lymph nodes (an indication that **inflammation** is affecting other parts of the body), are less common; and still others are extremely rare and frequently serious. It is worth emphasizing that *less than 5 percent* of people with RA develop the most serious consequences of the condition.

In this chapter the *less* common extra-articular features of RA are described. If you are experiencing any of these problems, *tell your doctor.*

Blood and Blood Vessels

How Does RA Affect the Blood?

Chapter 3 discussed the importance of testing the blood of a person with RA to determine whether that person has *anemia*. This blood disorder, which affects between one-half and two-thirds of all individuals with RA, is the condition that results when the number of red blood cells decreases notably. Anemia may develop as one of the consequences of longstanding inflammation, and its severity often reflects the activity of the arthritis. Called the *anemia of chronic disease,* this type of anemia usually improves when the arthritis is brought under control. In some situations, the drug *erythropoietin* can be administered intravenously to increase red blood cell production temporarily. This medication can be used in a presurgical situation, when an individual wants to donate his own blood for a scheduled surgery.

Another kind of anemia, called *iron deficiency anemia,* may develop as a side effect of taking anti-inflammatory drugs, which can irritate the stomach lining and cause minor (or, rarely, major) loss of blood. Anyone who develops iron deficiency anemia needs to be evaluated to determine whether he or she is losing blood from the stomach. This may mean examining the stool for blood or investigating the stomach using other techniques (an endoscopy or upper gastrointestinal series). It may be necessary to discontinue nonsteroidal anti-inflammatory drug (NSAID) therapy and to begin a course of stomach-healing medication (see Chapter 12).

Anemia may also develop as a component of an unusual complication of RA known as Felty's syndrome. This syndrome occurs in fewer than one of one hundred people who have longstanding RA. In addition to anemia and arthritis, people with Felty's syndrome develop an enlarged spleen and a decreased white blood cell count. A low white blood cell count means a reduction in the body's ability to fight infection and therefore means that infection is more likely to occur. Another complication of this syndrome is a decrease in the number of platelets in the blood, the blood cells involved in clotting. A low platelet count can be dangerous, because it carries the risk of excessive bleeding. Skin ulcerations and dark patches of skin are two other effects of Felty's syndrome.

Treatment for Felty's syndrome generally involves use of disease-modifying antirheumatic drugs (**DMARDs**). Occasionally, however, when medication proves ineffective and the person with Felty's syndrome experiences recurrent infections, the person's spleen must be removed surgically.

As noted above, individuals with RA do, rarely, develop a low platelet count (*thrombocytopenia*) as a result of Felty's syndrome. On the other hand, people with RA often have a *high* platelet count (*thrombocytosis*), a condition that is generally harmless and resolves with treatment of the arthritis.

What About the Blood Vessels?

Vasculitis (inflammation of blood vessels) is a rare complication of RA which generally affects individuals who have high levels of **rheumatoid factor** in their blood (the presence and level of rheumatoid factor can be detected by a blood test; see Chapter 3). Blood vessels may become inflamed when too many antibodies are being produced by the **plasma cells** in the blood. The **antibodies** stick to each other and form complexes, and those floating immune complexes sometimes deposit themselves on the blood vessel wall, causing inflammation within the blood vessel and limiting the flow of blood.

Depending on the size and location of the blood vessels involved, vasculitis can be a relatively minor problem or a more significant one. When small blood vessels leading to the skin are involved (particularly the skin in the lower legs), skin ulcers may develop. Splinterlike lesions around and under the fingernails may result when small blood vessels in that area are affected. These ulcers and lesions generally require only meticulous skin care (in addition to treatment of the underlying arthritis) to prevent secondary infection of the skin. Gently washing several times a day with a mild antiseptic soap (such as pHisoderm) and then thoroughly rinsing and drying the skin and applying sterile bandages is usually effective for this. Occasionally the advice and services of a **plastic surgeon** or **dermatologist** are useful.

When the blood vessels leading to the nerves are affected, numbness or weakness may result (this condition is known as *neuropathy*). More rarely, vasculitis involves the larger blood vessels that lead to internal organs. When nerves or internal organs are affected by vasculitis, very strong medications, including **corticosteroids** and cyclophosphamide, are used to treat the condition and prevent damage to nerves and organs.

Eyes and Mouth

About 15 percent of people with RA develop *sicca syndrome,* which causes them to have a dry mouth, dry eyes, or both. This syndrome produces inflammation in the tear glands, which in turn causes the eyes to become uncomfortably dry. Eyes that are not being bathed by sufficient quantities of tears can feel itchy or gritty or it may feel as if there is something in them. Occasionally, the eyelids become red and irritated.

A dry, windy climate or exposure to air conditioning can aggravate the symptoms, as can medications; certain kinds of cold medications, sleep-inducing medications, tranquilizers, and muscle relaxants can all increase eye dryness. If you are experiencing a problem with dry eyes, you may want to review your medications with your doctor. To help reduce the irritation of dry eyes, we also recommend the use of one of the many kinds of eye lubricants, or artificial tears, which are available both over the counter and by prescription.

Any other symptoms involving the eyes, such as pain, redness, or a change of vision, should immediately be brought to the attention of a physician. An **ophthalmologist** can examine the eyes to rule out the presence of either of the two other conditions that can affect the eyes in RA.

These are the rare conditions called **scleritis** and **episcleritis,** which may require treatment with topical corticosteroids or occasionally with medications taken by mouth. These serious complications of RA need to be monitored closely by an opthalmologist.

Dry mouth is another possible consequence of RA and is thought to be caused by inflammation of the salivary glands. Any of the medications mentioned above can exacerbate the problem of dry mouth, too.

For people who have a dry mouth, excellent oral hygiene is crucial, because a decrease in saliva can prompt tooth decay. Flossing the teeth and then gargling with an antiseptic mouthwash followed by thorough brushing with a tartar control toothpaste several times a day will help provide protection against decay. Ask your dentist about what products are right for you, and find out from your dentist whether fluoride treatments might be a good idea. It is also important to avoid lozenges and candies that contain sugar. Anyone who has a severe problem with mouth dryness or who experiences recurring swollen salivary glands should ask to be tested for primary Sjögren's syndrome, a condition that resembles RA.

Two new treatments are available that stimulate the salivary glands to produce saliva. These two medications are pilocarpine (Salagen) and cevimeline (Evoxac). Possible side effects of these medications include sweating and palpitations. Speak to your doctor if eye or mouth dryness is a severe problem for you.

Skin

People generally first notice skin nodules while dressing or bathing. They appear beneath the skin as small knots called rheumatoid **nodules,** and they occur in approximately one-quarter of people with established RA. They are more likely to appear in people who have rheumatoid factor than in people who don't have it (see Chapter 3).

Skin nodules often form close to joints, overlying areas that are susceptible to trauma or pressure, such as tendons or bony protrusions like the elbows, knuckles, or Achilles tendon. They often come and go in a pattern that follows the pattern of arthritis.

Rheumatoid nodules are benign (harmless) lumps that should not be confused with enlarged lymph nodes or tumors (which may or may not be harmless). The nodules are only bothersome when they press against internal body structures, interfere with the motion of a joint or tendon, or become infected. Rheumatoid nodules are not painful unless they are positioned in an area that is frequently traumatized, such as the heel tendon, which is rubbed by the back of the shoe. Rheumatoid nodules rarely appear in places other than the skin. On occasion they do appear in the lungs, heart, eyes, and vocal cords, but even in these places rheumatoid nodules seldom produce symptoms.

Rheumatoid nodules themselves do not merit special treatment unless they cause pain, decrease function, or become infected. Anyone who has rheumatoid nodules, however, should be considered for treatment with drugs that can produce remission, since the presence of nodules may indicate a more serious form of arthritis. Successful treatment with DMARDs can result in the resolution of nodules as well as improvement in arthritis. In a specific situation in which a particular nodule is causing structural problems, surgical removal is an option. Although removal of nodules for cosmetic reasons is generally discouraged, surgery is occasionally performed to improve appearance, too.

Nerves

Neuropathy, as stated above, is a rare complication resulting from inflammation in the blood vessels that lead to nerves. A more common form of neuropathy is one in which the person develops numbness or a burning sensation in a "glove-and-stocking" distribution without any obvious blood vessel disturbance. In most cases this second type of neuropathy improves with the effective treatment of arthritis.

Inflammation can create local pressure that squeezes or pinches nerves and thereby causes numbness or weakness. This nerve *compression* can result from swelling or from structural changes occurring in the joint. Nerves that travel near joints in the elbows and feet are sometimes compressed in RA, the most commonly pinched nerve being the median nerve that runs through the wrist. When the wrist becomes swollen, pressure increases in the joint, and the nerve becomes compressed. This causes numbness and tingling in the middle three fingers, a condition known as *carpal tunnel syndrome*. Carpal tunnel syndrome can also develop if the nerve becomes bent or kinked. Chronic inflammation sometimes changes the alignment of the wrist and so causes the nerve to deviate from its normal path. People who don't have RA can also develop carpal tunnel syndrome. It occurs most commonly in people who keep their wrists bent in the same position for long periods of time (such as people who work at computer terminals).

Wrist splints often help decrease symptoms of carpal tunnel syndrome in RA patients. Other means of decreasing inflammation, such as anti-inflammatory medications or **corticosteroid** injections into the wrist, are also helpful. If the symptoms of carpal tunnel syndrome are severe or persistent, surgery may be required.

Chest and Lungs

RA can produce breathing discomfort in two ways. The first occurs when the joints between the collar bones (*clavicles*) and chest bone (*sternum*) develop arthritis (see sternoclavicular joint in Figure 1). In this situation, which about 30 percent of people with RA develop, pain can occur when deep breaths are taken or when the shoulders are moved. The condition improves with treatment of the arthritis.

Between 10 and 20 percent of people with RA will at some point develop the other source of breathing discomfort, pleurisy, which causes pain deep in the chest and results from inflammation in the lining around the lungs (*pleura*). A complication of this inflammation is pleural effusion, or fluid around the lungs, which less than 5 percent of people with RA develop. This fluid generally produces few symptoms, and its presence is determined only by x-ray. Pleurisy and pleural effusion frequently improve with effective treatment of RA. If significant symptoms appear from pleural effusion, drainage of the fluid with a needle can be performed as an outpatient procedure. Temporary treatment with oral corticosteroids may be required.

Rarely, rheumatoid nodules develop in the lungs; these nodules are similar to those on the skin. They generally cause no symptoms and are diagnosed only by x-ray. The greatest difficulty is determining whether the nodule is a result of RA or another, unrelated, condition. A biopsy of the nodule may be required to determine its cause.

In only 1 or 2 percent of individuals with RA, a more serious lung problem known as **pneumonitis** arises. Cough and shortness of breath are indications that this problem may exist. Because the lung tissue is inflamed in pneumonitis, anti-inflammatory medications are administered promptly to decrease inflammation and prevent scarring (*fibrosis*).

Sometimes, but rarely, RA causes severe breathing difficulty, and the person requires hospitalization and urgent treatment to recover. If you ever experience difficulty breathing, be sure to consult your physician.

Vocal Cords

Another rare complication of RA is involvement of the joints of the vocal cords (*cricoarytenoid joints*). Usually there are no symptoms when this occurs, although some persons experience hoarseness, difficulty swallowing, a feeling of fullness in the throat, or pain radiating toward the ear. This complication is usually evaluated and treated by an ear, nose, and throat (*ENT*) doctor.

The Heart

The heart is seldom involved in RA, and when the heart is affected, most people experience no symptoms. When inflammation involves the membranous sac enclosing the heart (the pericardium), however, the person may experience symptoms similar to those of pleurisy. This condition is called *pericarditis*. In *rare* situations, a significant amount of fluid accumulates around the heart, a condition called *pericardial effusion*. This condition usually responds to **corticosteroids** and only rarely requires drainage of the fluid. Other parts of the heart are rarely involved in RA.

The Bones

People with RA are at higher risk of developing osteoporosis than is the general population. *Osteoporosis* is "thinning" of the bones or decreased "bone mass." Loss of bone makes a person more likely to sustain fractures. Researchers have recently discovered that inflammation plays a major role in the development of osteoporosis, even early in the course of RA. Pro-inflammatory **cytokines** (see Chapter 14) stimulate a protein called osteoprotegerin. This protein stimulates the activity of a group of cells called osteoclasts. Osteoclasts are well known for their ability to break down bone. It is normal for osteoclasts to cause some bone loss on a daily basis in everyone. This is balanced, however, by other cells, called osteoblasts, which build bone. During skeletal growth, the osteoblasts work harder than the osteoclasts, and bone growth occurs. In situations such as RA and menopause, the balance favors the osteoclasts, so bone loss occurs. Data are emerging that monitoring bone loss by bone densitometry (see "Bone density testing," Chapter 3) is increasingly important, particularly since there are now medications available to put the system back into balance and help restore good bone strength.

Women are at higher risk of osteoporosis than men are, because they start with less bone mass. At menopause, bone loss speeds up considerably. Men with RA are not spared completely from this condition, however. In addition to the direct effects of RA on bone, other changes can occur. Men with RA can have low levels of testosterone, which can cause additional bone loss and osteoporosis (Stafford et al. 2000).

Some arthritis medications can also increase the risk for osteoporosis. Corticosteroids are the most common cause of drug-induced bone loss. Life-style choices such as smoking and heavy alcohol use are toxic to bone. Also, being too sedentary and avoiding weight bearing exercises increase a person's risk of developing osteoporosis. A diet low in calcium and vitamin D also contributes to osteoporosis. (See Chapter 16 for osteoporosis treatments.)

Summary

Nonspecific symptoms of RA, including decreased appetite, fever, weight loss, and swollen lymph nodes, are relatively common and are not serious.

Red blood cell, white blood cell, and platelet counts can be affected by RA.

People with RA may experience symptoms related to dry eyes and mouth.

Rheumatoid nodules can occur over areas that receive pressure.

Serious involvement of the lungs, heart, eyes, nerves, and blood vessels can occur in RA, but these complications are rare.

People with RA are at higher risk of osteoporosis.

Many of these conditions improve as the arthritis is brought under control, whereas others require specific pharmaceutical or surgical treatment.

PART II

Coping with Rheumatoid Arthritis

·

CHAPTER 5

Coping Strategies

•

Life brings with it a series of changes, some of them predictable, others unpredictable. We encounter these changes, react to them, and adjust accordingly, often without being fully aware of what we're doing. Coping strategies that we develop along the way help us make effective adjustments so that we can grow with the resolution of each challenge and then move forward to face new experiences.

Because it brings a series of changes, life requires a series of adjustments. Those of you who are encountering the challenges posed by rheumatoid arthritis (RA) may know that physical, emotional, and financial changes may take place in your life during the coming years. You also know that there is no way to predict which changes will affect your life or when they will do so. Consider, though, that *now* may be the time to learn coping strategies that will enable you to adjust effectively to these changes, whatever they are and whenever they occur. Stress is the inevitable result when we fail to adapt, and therefore failure to make adjustments can make life even harder.

How will you address each of the changes RA brings to your life? How can you effectively meet the challenges that lie before you? You can explore various coping strategies and then develop and apply those that work best for you.

Coping strategies are neither complicated nor exotic; in fact, you have used them all of your life without realizing it. For example, consider that coping skills allowed you to make the transition from being a vulnerable youth to being a competent adult. You learned to cope with—and adjust to—being away from your family, earning your own money, buying groceries and preparing your own meals, and on and on.

Jonathan Swift once said, "Invention is the talent of youth, as judgment is of age." To cope effectively with RA, you must try to recapture the invention of youth and temper it with the judgment learned from experience. This involves developing new skills while improving upon old ones at the same time.

47

What's essential here is that you develop strategies that are effective for *you*, for it's been shown time and again that people benefit most from the strategies that they tailor for themselves, to fit their own needs. These strategies can be called into play over and over again as you approach each new challenge or crisis.

The following guidelines are provided to help you begin to design and adapt successful strategies for coping with RA; they can be helpful in showing you how to cope with other aspects of your life, too.

· Define and assess the problem.
· Set realistic goals and expectations.
· Develop methods for problem solving and negotiating.
· Use all available resources.
· Modify negative thoughts and behaviors.
· Be willing to reassess.

In the remainder of this chapter we will provide general information about what's involved in each of these guidelines. In Chapter 6 we suggest ways in which the strategies developed from these guidelines may help you cope with pain and fatigue. Chapter 7 describes how these strategies might be applied to help you handle your emotions and other people's reactions to your illness—because people sometimes respond in a way that is patronizing or hurtful, often without meaning to.

Define and Assess the Problem

To confront a problem, you first need to identify it. Although this may appear to be the obvious first step, it is a step that many people fail to take; and, once attempted, it is a step that often proves more difficult than people think.

As an example, suppose you are frustrated because you are having difficulty removing lids from jars. It may be that the physical act of removing the lids is your problem, but consider that this is easily remedied by calling upon other people to help you or by purchasing an assistive device (discussed in Chapter 8). If you ask for and obtain assistance from someone else or if you purchase an assistive device and are pleased with the results, then the physical act *was* the problem, and it has been solved. If using these appliances or asking for assistance makes you feel dependent and helpless, however, the problem is not your inability to remove the jar lids but your response to the need to seek assistance with a task that formerly you could perform easily on your own. In that case, identifying the problem becomes more difficult.

Before you can address it, you must recognize that a problem exists. Before you can solve a problem, you must *properly* identify it. As a general guideline, recognize that there will be times when you will need to think carefully about your own feelings to identify the problem properly.

Assessing a problem is different from identifying it. Assessment can best be carried out when you are as informed as possible about factual matters related to the problem. Being informed is particularly important if a physical limitation becomes a major problem, and that is one reason we recommend that you learn as much as you can about arthritis and its possible complications.

Consider this scenario: You have numbness in your fingers that wakes you up at night. Consequently, your sleep is disturbed, and you are constantly fatigued. If you think that feeling sleepy is your major problem, you are mistaken. Instead, numbness—the cause of your restless nights—is the origin of your difficulties. Rather than resorting to taking sleeping pills, a better course would be to pause to identify the problem properly and then to assess it. Seek more information. Dig deep. If you do, you will learn that inflammation in the wrists sometimes causes carpal tunnel syndrome, and you will also learn that wearing a wrist splint at night or taking an injection of a **corticosteroid** can make the numbness disappear, allowing more restful sleep. The combination of proper identification and appropriate information, then, can often lead to proper treatment and resolution of a problem.

There will definitely be times when you'll need to consult more than one source of information to assess a problem. When you are consulting a physician, for example, you may want to obtain an opinion from a different physician (a "second opinion") to satisfy yourself that you have enough information to assess and address the problem. Sometimes you'll want to talk with someone else just to get a fresh perspective on the problem. These are fine strategies, but a word of caution is in order here: It is important to avoid *overintellectualizing* a problem. If you spend all of your energy analyzing a problem, you will not move any closer to addressing it or solving it. It is easy to become obsessed with getting all the information, particularly with the availability of the Internet. Reading every available book and article on a subject or consulting numerous physicians ("doctor shopping") is an exaggerated version of a healthy analysis of a problem.

Set Realistic Goals and Expectations

When a problem is interfering with a given goal, you might ask yourself whether the goal is realistic *at that particular time*. If you determine that the goal is unrealistic, you may find that you needn't confront the problem you've been struggling with until later, when it may more easily be overcome. Or maybe, if you change your goal, you won't have to confront a particular problem at all. Do not let impossible expectations lock you into a no-win situation.

For example, if you begin an exercise program and you decide you want to be able to walk three miles by the third day, you are setting an unreasonable goal. If your house is a mess and you are not feeling well and you set a goal of having the house spotless by sunset, you are setting an unreasonable goal. Setting unreasonable goals sets you up to be disappointed and discouraged, and discouragement may make you give up on your exercise program or put off yet again getting a start on household chores. On the other hand, if you succeed in meeting an unrealistic goal, you may pay too large a price tomorrow.

A wiser plan is to divide the goal up into segments of small tasks that can be accomplished in steps. Not only will your ultimate goal stand a better chance of being accomplished (perhaps in a week rather than a day, or in four weeks rather than one), but you will also gain confidence in your capability to reach the other goals you set for yourself.

It is often helpful to make a contract with yourself composed of incremental assignments leading to the eventual goal. Success breeds success. Failure to attain an unrealistic expectation may make you resist trying again or afraid to try again. It may lower your confidence and self-esteem. On the other hand, when your self-expectations are in line with your capability, you are more likely to succeed.

A word about exercise plans (which are discussed in more detail in Chapters 9 and 10): If your goal is to improve your strength and endurance, don't become a weekend athlete. Instead, set daily exercise goals. Taking this approach will make it much more likely that you'll meet your goal.

Develop Methods for Problem Solving and Negotiating

You have identified a problem and established a reasonable goal. How do you proceed? How can you overcome barriers and reach your goal? You have several choices. You can:

· eliminate the problem,
· circumvent it,
· work with the obstacle, or
· modify the goal.

Each of these methods is effective in different situations. This is where imagination and creativity come into play.

Eliminating the Problem

After several weeks of having trouble rising from a chair because of arthritis in your knee, you discover that it is easier for you to get out of seats that are elevated. You then eliminate the problem by placing a firm, three-inch pillow in the seats of the chairs you will use. Your arthritis is still there, but the problem is solved.

A number of similar modifications can be made in your home and workplace environment to eliminate physical obstacles. In many ways, physical obstacles are the easiest to confront. But other kinds of problems can also be solved by eliminating the problem. Let your imagination expand the boundaries of your ideas.

Circumventing the Problem

Problem solving often involves working around a problem by, for example, changing habits and schedules. A common dilemma for people with RA is a workday that begins early, when morning stiffness restricts movement. One way around this problem would be to start the workday later if this can be arranged with your employer. Morning stiffness will not disappear, but no longer will it interfere with your work.

Working with the Obstacle

People often find that working with an obstacle that cannot be modified poses a serious challenge. Imagine, for example, that you are a trained data-entry person and you have arthritis in your fingers. You must work at the computer, but prolonged typing causes your fingers to hurt and cramp up. You enjoy your job and don't want to change it. To solve this problem you must first accept that the obstacle (arthritis in your finger joints) exists and then move on from there.

In this situation numerous options are available to someone who has developed coping strategies. One might be to take frequent breaks at regular intervals, before fatigue and pain develop. During breaks from the computer, you can perform other tasks that you have put aside for such times. You might want to keep a list of these tasks near the computer so you will always have other work to turn to, and you will not feel as if you are wasting time.

You can also call upon two interpersonal skills, communication and negotiation, and discuss with your supervisor your wish to assume other job responsibilities to replace some of the time you formerly spent at the computer. Expanding your job description to include other useful, but less physically demanding, responsibilities will balance your day. While you're making changes, you may also want to diversify your skills. For example, you might want to enroll in some courses that would prepare you to take on new tasks.

Work toward becoming more organized and imaginative. You may find that your productivity (and value to your employer) actually increases when you stretch yourself and your horizons.

Modifying the Goal

This is frequently a useful avenue for solving problems. Modifying the goal might involve changing your timetable for completion or dividing a task into mini-goals, as discussed above. Once you have established that your goal is realistic, you'll still need to reassess it and modify it along the way. It's this fine-tuning that will allow you to succeed in your endeavor.

Developing skills such as effective communication, organization, and scheduling is a crucial part of problem solving. Using these skills should not be considered overcompensation. Rather, using them will allow you to make the most of your potential. Armed with these skills, people with arthritis often become more productive in every aspect of their lives.

Utilize All Available Resources

People are often surprised to discover how much inner strength they can muster when they are faced with adversity. The truth, however, is that we all depend on our inner resources to get through each day. Intangibles such as courage, optimism, and faith, as well as our creativity and skill in problem solving, are at our disposal to help us overcome hurdles.

You don't have to depend solely on your own inner strength, however. Family, friends, health care professionals, arthritis support groups, religious groups, social service organizations, and vocational rehabilitation centers—any and all of these can provide an invaluable source of support and encouragement. Although some of these people are trained and skilled in helping, others who are willing to help will need some guidance to know what they are to do. Access to resources has never been better.

Although you may be hesitant to seek outside help, you might consider that utilizing the special skills and support of other people is a coping strategy that benefits you *and* them. By helping you to help yourself, their assistance may allow you to retain your independence. Ironically, their lives will also be richer, since they have been able to contribute something to someone who needed their help.

Modify Negative Thoughts and Behaviors

When a new problem develops, it is tempting to indulge in negative thinking. After all, negative thinking is a part of human nature, and we all fall victim to it on occasion. Because RA is a chronic condition and the problems it poses often appear overwhelming, it is only natural that negative thoughts will occupy you from time to time.

Conversely, it can be hard work to maintain a positive attitude. When we're in the middle of a thunderstorm, it is difficult to focus on the sun hidden behind the clouds. While acknowledging the difficulty of maintaining a positive attitude, let it be said: *Persistent negative thinking is harmful.* Persistent negative thinking can be our worst enemy. For one thing, negativism is often irrational in that it is based on emotions more than on facts. Focusing on negative thoughts usually makes us feel worse, and negative thoughts can lead us to take negative actions, alienating the people we love and need. Finally, negative thinking does not lead us to develop solutions to problems or help us to accomplish goals. In other words, it doesn't lead us to where we want to be.

Try to be vigilant about negative thinking: When you notice yourself thinking negative thoughts, stop yourself and redirect your thoughts. Tell yourself what you need to hear to stop these thoughts. For example, you might ask yourself, "How does this thought help me?" Or you can say to yourself, "Stop this useless rubbish"; "Enough of this negative thinking"; "These ideas are getting me nowhere." Perhaps the words that work for you are as simple as "Cut that out." In fact, sometimes if you become a little angry with (or even insulting to) yourself, you can "snap out" of negativity with relative ease.

Once you recognize the thought as negative, look at it. What caused you to have this thought? Did this thought help you? Hurt you? Then modify the thought into something constructive. This strategy, called *positive reappraisal,* can be an extremely useful tool in coping with any chronic illness.

Here are some examples of positive reappraisal:

Negative thought: "I can't do this."
Modified thought: "This will be a challenge, but I'll try to do it one step at a time."
Self-message: I am innovative and capable.

Negative thought: "I can't play ball with Billy like other fathers can with their kids."
Modified thought: "I'll show Billy the antique cars at the auction and we'll have a great time together."

Self-message: I have a lot to offer, and others enjoy my company.

Negative thought: "I'll just be in their way."
Modified thought: "We always have a good time together."
Self-message: They love me, not my joints.

Negative thought: "I don't even want to get out of bed."
Modified thought: "I'll feel so much better after my nice warm shower."
Self-message: I can help myself.

Negative thought: "My boss is a heartless jerk."
Modified thought: "I'll talk to my boss about ways that I can be more effective in my job."
Self-message: I am on the way to becoming a more valued employee.

Negative thought: "This is all my fault."
Modified thought: "I'd rather not have arthritis, but I will learn to work with it."
Self-message: Many good people have RA. I am a good person and I did not cause myself to have RA.

Negative thought: "I'll never get ahead."
Modified thought: "I am really becoming organized."
Self-message: I can develop skills I never had before.

Negative thought: "No one helps me; I'll just do it myself."
Modified thought: "I will develop a chore list for the kids and discuss why it's necessary that we work together as a family."
Self-message: Communication is essential; asking for help is okay.

Negative thought: "I will end up in a wheelchair."
Modified thought: "Most people with RA live normal lives, and I will too."
Self-message: Facts, not emotions, should control my thoughts.

Finally, it's important to remember that you only compound your troubles if you feel guilty about your negative thoughts. Everyone has them. You simply need to learn to redirect them and not let them control you.

A good mental attitude is extremely powerful. It can't eliminate the arthritis, but it can definitely improve your ability to function, mentally and physically. Positive thoughts can provide you with sanctuary in even the most troublesome of situations. You can concentrate on treasuring each of your blessings rather than toting up all of your disappointments. This will fortify you and make you a person with whom other people will want to spend time.

Be Willing to Reassess

RA is unpredictable and often appears to follow a random and uncertain course. The frustration of this uncertainty can in itself be a significant impediment to effective coping. Why? Because you cannot predict when you will have a bad day. Nor can you predict when you will have a good day. This makes planning ahead difficult, and it means there will be times when plans made will become plans changed.

People with RA often feel as if they are on an emotional roller coaster: Just when things appear to be under control, a flare-up of arthritis occurs and changes everything. A life that is full of "ups and downs" is difficult to deal with, but flexibility—learning to make *adjustments to changes*—can help you avoid becoming discouraged. You will need to remain flexible, and you will need to adjust your expectations and plans regularly.

The key to flexibility is expecting and accepting unpredictability. If you accept the unpredictable nature of RA, you won't feel quite so disappointed when your arthritis acts up. Ask yourself, "Am I better prepared to deal with this flare-up than I was a month ago?" Most likely you are. You will learn how to deal with each flare-up without allowing it to knock you down. Many people adjust to the unpredictability by backing up their scheduled plans with contingency arrangements. Many people use coping strategies to solve new problems as they occur. These people don't passively let life happen to them; they take steps to prepare themselves for what life brings their way. Learning and perfecting strategies for coping with change is the successful antidote for the unpredictability of RA.

For More Information

The Arthritis Self-Management Program was developed in 1979, under the auspices of the Arthritis Foundation, by Kate Lorig, D.P.H., and James Fries, M.D. This course emphasizes developing self-efficacy skills. To locate a self-help course in this program, contact your local Arthritis Foundation chapter.

Out of the Arthritis Self-Management Program came a book: *The Arthritis Helpbook: A Tested Self-Management Program for Coping with Arthritis and Fibromyalgia,* 5th edition, by Kate Lorig and James Fries (Cambridge, Mass.: Perseus Publishing, 2000).

CHAPTER 6

Coping with Pain and Fatigue

•

For the person who has rheumatoid arthritis (RA), pain and fatigue may be overwhelming at times, so much so that they leave the person feeling anxious and depressed as well as in pain and tired. But both pain and fatigue come and go, and their severity changes as well. (In fact, pain and fatigue are often most limiting during the early stages of RA.)

There's no question that pain and fatigue are complicated symptoms that are frequently difficult to explain and understand. Like other aspects of RA, however, pain and fatigue are most effectively controlled when they are understood. For this reason, the person who makes the effort and takes the time to learn the causes, significance, and aggravating factors of his or her pain and fatigue is much more likely to be able to manage these symptoms.

Pain

The pain of RA may be the most burdensome feature of your illness, especially when pain interferes with your ability to function as you once did. Because RA is a chronic condition, you may wonder whether you'll always suffer this much pain. The answer is No!

What Is Pain?

A very simple explanation of pain is that it begins as a message from stimulated nerve endings (or pain receptors); this message is transmitted from the nerves to the spinal cord to the brain, where the message is interpreted as pain. Irritation, inflammation, or injury can activate the pain receptors. Even when the message is painful, we have to be thankful for it, because it can prevent a more severe injury. For example, when you accidentally touch a hot stove, stimulated pain receptors in your fingertips send a message to your brain that a dangerous situation exists—*tissue is being dam-*

aged. After your brain interprets the signal, it quickly sends a message back to the hand: "That hurts. . . . Pull away!" Pain can protect us!

The circuitry from the painful stimulus to the brain and back is incredibly intricate. In 1965 Ronald Melzack and Patrick Wall proposed the *gate theory of pain,* which helps us understand just how complex pain perception is. They suggested that there is a "gate" located in the spinal cord which can be opened or closed under various situations. According to these researchers, when the gate is open, pain messages can pass through to the brain (although only a limited amount of sensory information can pass through the gate at one time). Interestingly enough, the body can send messages that compete with each other; one message can send a pain signal, and another can effectively close the gate to prevent that signal from being received.

If you have ever stubbed your toe or banged your elbow you have experienced this phenomenon. Once you begin rubbing the affected area (as most of us will do under the circumstances!) you send a message that competes with the pain message. This instinctive reaction to pain works because the sensation of rubbing is transmitted to the spinal cord through nerve fibers that are larger than the fibers through which pain travels to the spinal cord. The message of rubbing is dispatched rapidly to the spinal cord, whereas the message of pain travels slowly, through small nerve fibers. Reaching the spinal cord before the pain message, the comforting, rubbing message blocks out the slower, sharp pain signal and prevents it from reaching the brain. Without knowing it, you have closed the pain gate by your instinctive reaction.

The brain also appears to have its own mechanisms for decreasing acute pain; that is, in times of need, the brain apparently has the capacity to send signals to close the gate. This capacity to close the gate is extremely powerful. We have all heard accounts of someone running into a burning building to save a child, for example. Although that person gets burned, he or she continues the quest to save a life. Or what about the football player who crosses the goal line on a broken or sprained limb? These individuals often relate that they felt very little pain during the experience. Why?

The theory is that the body produces its own morphinelike substances, endorphins and enkephalins, and that these protective chemicals may be responsible for closing the pain gate in the situations described above. Stories such as these make us appreciate how powerful the brain can be in overcoming pain.

Chronic pain, which can be nearly continuous or unremitting, is very different from the transient and acute pain described in the examples above. It differs both scientifically and emotionally. The brain can overcome chronic pain, too, although different processes are required for it to do so.

Pain and Your Emotions

Researchers, physicians, and patients all know that the degree of pain experienced from RA is not always proportional to the amount of inflammation present. From this fact we must infer that some people perceive pain more intensely than others. How intensely you experience pain is linked in part to your emotions and to your understanding of what the pain *signifies*.

Pain that follows war injuries is a well-documented example of how a person's perception of pain can be affected by the *meaning* that person attaches to it. In these instances, people who are severely wounded in battle often report feeling little or no pain after the injury. Perhaps this is because the injury signifies their freedom to return home. Or maybe their pain reminds them of the courage they displayed while fighting for a cause. On the other hand, a senseless and arbitrary automobile accident with a similar degree of injury will usually cause greater emotional and physical pain.

Because the pain of RA has different personal *significance* for each individual, it only follows that the pain will be experienced differently by each person. The person for whom each twinge of pain symbolizes loss of function and control will probably vigilantly monitor and focus on his pain and may end up feeling that pain more intensely than someone who learns to view pain as a message alerting him to modify his actions and prevent joint damage. Sometimes a positive attitude really can improve your condition.

Emotions also play a remarkable role in the perception of pain. Does that mean that the pain is all in your head? Certainly not! It is in our joints and muscles. But your emotions can intensify or lessen the perception of that painful stimulus from the joints and muscles. People who feel confident, organized, and in control often experience less pain. Those who are fearful or depressed suffer much higher levels of pain.

Emotions can also increase pain directly. To illustrate this phenomenon, consider one of the most common sources of pain in RA, muscle spasm. Muscles that are continuously tight and do not relax adequately can be very painful. Joint pain can often promote reflex muscle spasm, or tension. When the muscle contracts and squeezes around painful joints, they become even more painful. In addition to joint pain, here are some other notorious sources of muscle tension:

· stress   · anxiety   · fear   · depression
· poor sleep patterns   · fatigue   · isolation

Do any of these conditions sound familiar? The truth is, we all encounter these conditions in our day-to-day lives. Many of them are unavoidable.

Depression, fear, and other emotional reactions to life events (and to life in general) can provoke muscle tension, as can poor sleep patterns. In RA as in other conditions, these factors often trigger a vicious cycle of pain which is difficult to break.

What Is the Pain Message in RA?

We've stated that pain is a signal or message. What exactly is that message in the case of RA? In RA, inflammation that occurs in the joints can irritate nerve endings in the joint lining (synovium), capsule, and ligaments. This inflammation leads to swelling within the joints, which causes these same structures to become stretched. Inflammation causes pain, and that pain is intensified by swelling. Pain from joints that are highly inflamed (warm, swollen, and tender) sends the following messages: (1) Respect your pain. (2) Slow down, you're overdoing it. (3) Protect and rest your joints until the inflammation subsides.

Decreasing Pain

Just because pain is a valued signal doesn't mean you have to suffer through it without trying to decrease its intensity. After all, pain is exhausting! The first step in decreasing the intensity of pain is accepting that pain exists in your present life. This doesn't mean that you should surrender to a painful existence; it simply means that you must accept the fact that your joints are painful *today* and that you'll need to direct your energies toward getting through today. If you are filled with regrets about the past and fears of the future, you are fighting the presence of pain in your life. Regret and fear are wasted emotions that create feelings of guilt, blame, and anxiety, and these cause you further pain *today*. It is true but ironic that accepting pain is the first step in decreasing it.

Next, recognize pain as being a very personal experience. Understanding that each person has a unique awareness of his or her pain is critical, because effective strategies for combatting pain will differ for each person. You will need to take responsibility for your experience of pain, from how you perceive it to how you handle it. This does not mean accepting the blame for having RA. Rather, it means *not* viewing pain as an outside force that is directing you; don't allow your pain to have that much power! Instead, view pain as a force over which you can exert some control. This will mean assessing the source of your pain, the conditions that worsen it, your perception of it, and options that will allow *you* to direct *it*.

Once you have accepted the presence of pain in your life and taken responsibility for your unique experience of it, how can you begin to control it? You can select any or all of the following options.

Define and assess your problem. To use this coping tool (first discussed in Chapter 5), think about what is causing your pain. Trace your daily activities to determine whether some specific activity may be aggravating your unusually painful joints. If you identify such an activity, plan ahead to modify it in the future. The following examples may help you to find the cause of your pain and develop methods to alleviate and control it.

1. Pain in the morning. Morning stiffness and pain are usually related to inflammation. Setting your alarm clock to go off one hour before you need to get out of bed can help. Keep your medications at bedside, and take them then. An electric blanket can be useful in warming up the bed and your joints. Perform your gentle range of motion exercises in bed to loosen up your joints before getting up.

After you have risen, go directly from bed to a warm shower or bath (maybe someone else can draw the bath ahead of time). In other words, ease into morning slowly, and give your joints ample time to loosen up.

2. Pain after sitting (called **gelling**). This pain is also caused by inflammation in the joints. Gelling can usually be alleviated by taking frequent stretch breaks during prolonged stationary periods.

3. Pain after exercise. If pain persists for more than two hours after exercising, you have overextended yourself. Analyze your exercise—distance walked, number of repetitions done, footwear worn, etc.—and review your exercise program with your doctor or therapist.

4. Pain with specific activities. Some examples: twisting lids, getting into the shower, styling your hair, bending down to pick things up, carrying objects, making love. All of these activities can be modified to limit joint stress. (More about this later.)

The general approach here is to analyze painful activities, either by taking mental notes or keeping a diary, and then to modify them.

Protect your inflamed joints. Protecting inflamed joints from excessive stress will decrease pain. In Chapter 8 we discuss the use of splints and describe techniques for avoiding stressful joint actions. Your **occupational therapist,** an expert in this area, will be an invaluable source of information to you. Skills for protecting your joints require only a little extra time, and once you see how effective they are, you undoubtedly will make them an automatic part of your daily life.

Improve your muscle health. The two methods of improving your muscle health are to (1) reduce muscle tension and (2) increase muscle strength. We have described how muscle tension contributes to joint pain. Certainly, warm baths or showers, warm compresses, relaxation techniques, gentle massage, imagery techniques, adequate rest and sleep, and tailored exercises will be of great value in reducing muscle tension. You can learn to do many of these treatments for yourself.

Increasing muscle strength is an excellent way to take stress (and thus pain) away from joints by providing increased structural support. A **physical therapist** trained in arthritis treatment can instruct you in exercise programs designed to increase muscle strength. (Physical therapists can assist you with other techniques for effectively reducing pain; electrical stimulation, ultrasound, and hydrotherapy are examples.)

Close the pain gate. Emotional factors are as crucial as physical factors in creating your experience of pain. What methods can you employ to decrease the transmission of pain through the pain gate?

1. Utilize distraction. An enjoyable pastime is always an excellent means of distracting your mind from pain. Watching a favorite television show or videotape, going out to the theater to see a movie or play, reading a book, telephoning an old friend, taking a college course, exploring new hobbies—all of these activities can take your mind off your joints. Look for fun. Laughter is a great analgesic (pain reliever) and a muscle relaxant that has no adverse effects. The prospect of having fun might seem inconceivable, because you feel so miserable, but if you pursue enjoyable activities, you *will* have fun.

2. Change your beliefs about pain. There are two ways to accomplish this. One is to view your pain scientifically as being a valued signal that provides a protective function for your joints. Viewed this way, pain is less likely to foster fear, anxiety, or depression.

Another technique is **imagery.** When your pain is overwhelming, try using visual imagery to change your view of it. Here are two examples you can experiment with. Begin each of them by sitting or lying down and then closing your eyes and taking a few long, deep breaths.

Example 1. Concentrate on your warm, painful joints, likening them to an uncomfortably hot, blazing fire. Imagine yourself slowly moving farther and farther from the flames, feeling less heat. Or imagine a cool, summer shower gently extinguishing the fire and the pain.

Example 2. Think of the pain throbbing in your knees as being like a team of horses, galloping out of control. Imagine yourself controlling the reins, slowing the horses down to a gentle pace. Then visualize a pleasant ride through the countryside, breathing in the fresh air, enjoying the surroundings.

In each of these examples, you are creating healing images to counteract the painful ones. If you can become involved in your images, your body will respond as if they were real. Muscles will relax, heart rate and breathing rate will decrease, and pain can subside.

3. Address your stress, anxiety, depression, and fatigue. Remember that these symptoms and emotions lower your pain threshold by opening the pain gates and creating muscle tension.

Minimize inflammation. As mentioned above, learning to avoid activities that increase your joint inflammation is crucial, but if you do find that you have some postactivity inflammation, try applying cold packs (or wrapped "blue ice") to the warm joints for 20 minutes. Always wrap ice and other sources of extreme cold in a towel before placing them next to your skin.

There are several approaches to controlling inflammation. Most notably, your physician will prescribe medications for controlling inflammation. Nonsteroidal anti-inflammatory drugs (**NSAIDs**) are commonly used to decrease pain and inflammation over a period of days. Other medications, such as **DMARDs**, are intended to induce more sustained improvement, but they work over weeks to months, by inducing control of the rheumatoid process.

Narcotics mask pain without changing the underlying condition, and so your physician may be reluctant to prescribe large amounts of these medications for you. This is not because he or she is heartless; rather, totally masking pain would not be in your joints' best interests. Remember, pain can provide a valuable message; if you don't feel pain, you will not receive your body's warning signal, and you may overexert yourself and cause serious damage to your joints.

Another reason your physician will want to avoid having you use narcotics on a long-term basis is the addictive potential of these medications. If you develop a physical requirement for these medications, you may find that you have relinquished control over your body and given it to the prescribing physician. This places you in the uncomfortable position of having to convince your doctor that you are in severe pain so that he or she will continue to prescribe narcotics for you.

If you can use your mind's capacity to control pain, *you* will be in charge.

Fatigue

You may find that fatigue is the most incapacitating feature of RA. Fatigue can limit your concentration and ability to function, so that even mustering sufficient energy to care for your family or to participate in social activities—much less to deal with the responsibilities of the workplace—can be difficult. The normal demands of everyday living can sometimes appear overwhelming to the person who is chronically tired.

Sometimes the fatigue and loss of energy which result from RA are severe. In fact, many people think that there must be something else wrong with them in addition to arthritis because they cannot believe that arthritis alone can affect their energy so drastically.

Fatigue may be unpredictable, and so it can interfere with plans you've made. You may feel exasperated or frightened by this loss of control over your energy level. Tiredness also contributes to depression, anxiety, and pain; remember, fatigue increases pain in your joints. You need to know what you can do to alleviate this pervasive symptom.

Why Am I So Tired?

Fatigue or decreased energy in RA can be caused by the condition itself or by emotional upheaval, pain, lack of sleep, and general lack of physical fitness. Remember, RA is a systemic condition that can affect more than just the joints. The **anemia** that sometimes results from the condition, for example, can contribute to fatigue. Also, fatigue may be a consequence of inflammatory substances (**cytokines**) in the blood; this fatigue may come on suddenly, early in the course of the disease, and may resemble the tiredness that accompanies a virus or flu. Effective control of RA through appropriate medications will lessen cytokine-induced fatigue.

Your emotions alone can exhaust you; think of how tired you feel after you've had a particularly emotional experience. Pain can be emotionally and physically exhausting, too; and when pain is combined with anxiety and tension, limited energy reserves can be depleted easily. Depression can amplify fatigue. It's easy to see that effectively controlling pain, anxiety, and depression is an important factor in controlling fatigue.

Obviously, fatigue can be the result of inadequate sleep. Researchers at Chapel Hill, North Carolina, recently reported that sleep disruption appears to be a common consequence of arthritis (Jordan et al., 2000). For people with RA, painful joints, tight muscles, fear, and anxiety frequently interfere with the ability to get a good night's sleep.

Finally, when people have had RA for a while, they may get out of condition. This loss of physical fitness may be a consequence of decreased activity, and it produces a different form of exhaustion.

Controlling Fatigue

Get adequate rest. Individuals with RA require more rest than they did before they developed the condition. Adequate rest takes many forms, including physical, emotional, and "local" rest (described below).

Getting adequate sleep is imperative, because sleep provides healing to the body and the mind. We recommend ten hours of sleep daily, particularly during periods when the arthritis has flared up. You may prefer to sleep eight hours at night and take two one-hour naps during the day. If getting adequate sleep proves difficult, ask your doctor to recommend or prescribe pain or sleeping medications to help you.

Actual sleep is not the only way to rest physically and emotionally. Taking a fifteen- or twenty-minute break in the morning and afternoon can also make an incredible difference in productivity. Learning and performing stress reduction and relaxation techniques during tense times may be particularly beneficial (see Chapter 7). During these breaks try to relax your mind and body. If you can manage to lie down with your feet elevated, you'll increase the benefits of the break. Deep breathing exercises can also markedly reduce fatigue, particularly if combined with meditation. Taking prescribed breaks routinely each day may allow you to avoid the severe exhaustion that occurs when you become overly fatigued.

From time to time it's a good idea to reflect on the day's activities. Think about what you did during the day and when you felt most tired. This review will allow you to schedule your rest breaks strategically, which will help you avoid becoming overtired. If necessary, discuss these recommendations with your employer; he or she will probably agree that this is time well spent. It is to everyone's benefit for you to retain your energy so you can be as efficient and productive as possible.

Local rest means resting specific parts of the body. Getting local rest will help you protect your joints from undue stress; this can be achieved by wearing splints, which can be fabricated to protect the wrists and hands, and by using techniques designed to reduce joint stress (these are discussed in detail in Chapter 8).

Set priorities. Your energy is most limited when your RA is flaring, and at these times it may not be possible for you to do everything you would like to do or feel that you *should* do. At these times you need to be honest with yourself about what you can and cannot do. Start by setting priorities. Make lists of things to do, and then prioritize those things. Decide to do first what absolutely must be done, and cross out everything that has the word *should* connected to it: "I *should* iron my dress." Instead, select a dress to wear that doesn't need ironing, even if you just wore it last week. Being fashion conscious is a low priority if it is at the expense of energy that you don't have. "I should do some dusting tonight." The dust isn't going anywhere! Put that task aside until you have more energy, or consider assigning that task to someone else.

After you have thrown out the shoulds, divide the remaining tasks into steps. Discard the all-or-nothing philosophy. (Cleaning day—"I must do all my cleaning in one day so my whole house is clean at one time"—is an example of an all-or-nothing item you may find on your list.) Do a little each day, and eventually it will all get done.

Plan ahead. A little organization and planning will save you vast amounts of wasted energy. For example, an efficient work space is extremely important. In your place of employment, store all the equipment that you generally need within easy reach and at a convenient height. Put things in their place, and know where things are kept. This way you won't waste energy looking for things or getting up frequently to retrieve something. Avoid clutter both at work and at home, and ask others to help you with this.

At home, store necessities for each task near the place where the task is performed. For example, store the wash detergent with the laundry basket, washer, and dryer. (Incidentally, asking family members to bring their dirty clothes to—and collect their clean ones from—the laundry area means that each person expends a little energy rather than one person expending a lot.)

For you, effective planning might involve participating in more bulk activities. For instance, cooking bulk quantities on the weekend is a great idea. Making a large pan of lasagna or batch of chili and freezing portions for future use can save a lot of energy during a busy week. And if you wake up not feeling very well, you can take a package from the freezer for dinner later. Keeping convenience foods on hand for bad days is another good idea.

Bulk shopping can be useful, too. Once a month take someone shopping with you and purchase staple items that you know you'll need for the month: sugar, flour, condiments, paper goods, cereal. That way you'll only need to shop more frequently for perishables, and your shopping load will be lighter. Avoid purchasing items in industrial size containers, however, because these will put stress on your hands and wrists (or, if you prefer to buy goods in these large containers, make plans to divide them up into smaller portions).

What about energy for social outings? You may be avoiding all social events, fearing that you won't have enough energy or that you'll hold everyone else back. There are *some* activities you will temporarily need to avoid when your energy level is very low. These activities include all-or-none outings that don't allow time for adequate rest breaks (large group walking tours are notorious for this). You shouldn't have to push yourself in an effort to keep up. If you must decline a social invitation, be sure to let your friends know that you are still interested in future activities and want to be included. Your task will be to help organize activities with your family and friends which will allow for rest. Then remember to rest adequately the day before a planned activity. Only you know your own limitations. If you take an interest in outside activities you'll find that loved ones can be extremely flexible. After all, it makes them feel bad when you can't participate. So, get involved.

Avoid wasting energy. We waste a lot of energy during the course of a day, so part of effective energy conservation involves asking questions such as, "Is there an easier way to accomplish this?" Simple changes, such as taking the elevator instead of walking the stairs, can save energy. Using carts to carry equipment or utensils even for small distances saves energy and wear and tear on hand and wrist joints. Sitting down to do activities that you usually perform standing can reduce knee and hip fatigue. Consider this: Do you *really* need to stand to wash dishes or shave or fix your hair? Break habits! Get a high stool, sit, and relax while you perform these necessary tasks.

You can also avoid wasting energy by establishing a step-by-step routine for tasks you undertake regularly. With proper planning, you can reduce the steps in some tasks and combine the steps in other tasks, and perhaps you can even eliminate some steps. Make each task as simple as possible.

Pace yourself. Pacing involves developing guidelines for energy expenditure. The amount of activity that precipitates fatigue among individuals is extremely variable, so you are the only one who can set guidelines for yourself. As a general rule, however, it's a good idea to alternate energy-intensive activities with more relaxing ones throughout the day. This kind of balance added to your routine can prevent excessive fatigue.

Almost everyone with RA tries to "catch up" on days when they feel well, but using good days to their maximum has its drawbacks. Try not to overutilize those days, since doing so may result in a flare-up of your arthritis.

Division of labor. Do not try to do everything by yourself. Instead, divide chores among several people to help lighten the workload. If you live with a partner or children, your job may be easier. If your children are old enough, set up schedules and jobs. It is simple to provide incentives to convince your children to help you, since there is always some small reward that they can earn. Helping with household chores is a great lesson in responsibility as well.

If you live alone, the challenge is greater, although not impossible. Meeting the challenge involves family or friends or neighbors who might be willing to help you. If you can think of something that you can do for them in return, you won't be so reluctant to ask for assistance. For example, many young couples have difficulty finding affordable baby sitters whom they can depend on and trust. When presented with the opportunity for a free Saturday night, they will probably view your request that they mow your lawn or vacuum your carpets as a great bargain. Everyone wins! Your imagination sets the limits. If you have special skills, use them in exchange for help. Obviously, many people will be happy to help you for nothing in return. The important thing is for *you* to feel good about asking for help.

Get in shape. Being out of condition will almost always result in fatigue, and having RA means that it will be more difficult to stay in top condition. When your arthritis flares up, you have to rest your joints and muscles. This in turn leaves your body out of condition.

With appropriate medical therapy, the inflammation in your joints will eventually decrease. At this point you will need to get more involved in an exercise program. (See Chapter 10 for information about aerobic exercises that will increase your conditioning and help you get back in shape.)

Make use of medical therapy. Medications are useful in the long-term control of fatigue. As disease-modifying antirheumatic drugs (DMARDs) begin working to control your RA, fatigue will also lessen. Anemia will also improve with the control of arthritis. Use the skills above to cope with fatigue until your arthritis is brought under control. Then continue using them to make your life easier, more convenient, and more fun.

For More Information

Two helpful pamphlets, "Managing Your Fatigue" and "Managing Your Pain," are available from the Arthritis Foundation (1330 W. Peachtree St., Atlanta, Ga. 30309; 1-800-283-7800).

CHAPTER 7

Coping with Emotions—
Yours and Everyone Else's

•

It is easy to see how this change in your life can affect the way you deal with yourself and with others. You may worry, at first, about how your friends and family will respond when they notice the changes in you. Or you may be surprised at the intensity of your own emotional responses to rheumatoid arthritis (RA). Many of the emotions triggered by RA are those we would rather not experience. Eventually, however, you and all of the people around you will learn how to cope with RA, including the accompanying emotions.

The feelings we have about the changes taking place in our lives are completely natural, but that doesn't mean we have to let them control us. For example, we know that a person who is plagued by negative thoughts and feelings is much more likely to feel tired than a person whose thoughts are optimistic. Persistent negative emotions drain human energies. If you are overcome by negativity, then you are reducing the amount of energy that is available to you for activities such as dining out, swimming, painting—all of the things you *like* to do.

One of the emotions you may experience is grief; you may initially grieve because you have arthritis. This is nothing to be ashamed of because everyone grieves over losses. Most people want others to share their grief too, and they find that this helps them overcome their sense of loss. Learning to understand your feelings and cope with them will help you in all aspects of your life. On the other hand, if you let your feelings control *you*, they may affect your ability to cope with arthritis and every other aspect of your daily living. You can face these emotions head on and redirect your energy toward improving your condition.

Anger

Why shouldn't you be angry? You probably have found it necessary to give up activities that you truly enjoy. Your days are more difficult and complicated than they used to be. It seems that no one really understands the pain and frustration you're experiencing. You're frustrated with your doctor because your recovery is not as speedy as you would like it to be. These thoughts are all valid, and they would leave anyone feeling angry.

People respond to anger in several ways—and in different ways at different times. They may direct their anger inward, for example; people often blame themselves for their situation and suffer feelings of guilt as a result. Or they may direct their anger toward other people. Sometimes anger is suppressed entirely. Bottled up anger raises blood pressure, increases muscle tension and pain, and drains precious energy reserves.

Some people are angry and don't know it. Their anger is so well disguised that they fail to recognize it. Each of the following thoughts, or self-messages, contains a disguised element of anger:

"I'm just going to finish this project at my own pace, and if he doesn't like it, that's his problem."
"Why would I want to go golfing, anyway?"
"What does *she* know about arthritis?"
"He's just helping me because he feels guilty."
"I'm just not going to take that worthless pill."
"I should have stopped smoking and exercised more often."

People who make statements or have thoughts such as these are angry about their arthritic condition and the havoc it is creating in their lives. One of the dangers of unrecognized anger is that it is often turned against other people, in the form of casting blame, harboring resentment, or engaging in passive-aggressive behavior. This response hurts people who really care about you and only want to help you.

Managing Anger

The first step in dealing with any emotion is to recognize it. Once you recognize that you're angry, you'll have an easier time managing it. The coping strategies described in Chapter 5 can help you deal with anger.

First, *define and assess the source of anger*. The people in the following stories have recognized that they are angry, and they have identified the source of their anger.

Janice is angry because arthritis is interfering with her work. She's always been a competent and respected employee, and she hates the way her arthritis has changed her previously successful work routine.
Margaret is angry because her family doesn't understand the emotional and physical chaos she is going through. She feels that there is a lack of help and encouragement in her home. She works all day and comes home feeling too tired to perform simple household tasks.

Ken is frustrated and angry about the unfairness of having RA. He has always exercised, eaten right, and kept himself in excellent physical condition. He is angry that despite his good habits, he has arthritis. Friends who were not nearly as health conscious as he remain unscathed. "Why me? What did I do wrong?" he continues to ask himself.

Second, *set realistic goals and expectations.* Arthritis is interfering with Janice's work, and she's angry. Why? Is it possible that she's expecting too much from herself? Or are other people expecting more from her than she can provide at this time? It seems that Janice expects to be able to continue performing her job exactly as she's always done it, and she's frustrated because she can't. It also seems that she is stubbornly attached to her routine and has not accepted the changes in her capabilities. Janice needs to redefine her expectations. She needs to consider whether her routine is really that important and whether her schedules really need to be so rigidly defined.

Does Margaret expect her family to know automatically how she is feeling simply because they love her? Do they even have any idea of how they can best help her? Should they be able to sense that she is really angry about having arthritis, or are they receiving signals that she is angry at them? Are Margaret's expectations of her family reasonable?

People with RA have done nothing to bring this condition upon themselves, and so a person with RA might easily view the situation as being unfair. Two facts are significant here. First, RA, like many other conditions, is neither fair nor just. Second, unfairness as a source of anger is difficult to resolve. It will never be possible for Ken to view his condition as being fair. He may try to "make things even" by making his friends feel as badly as he does about it, but he won't ever be able to make things fair in his own estimation. Any expectation of fairness is likely to result in frustration and anger. It seems that the only way around this, again, is to *change your expectations.* Don't expect things to be fair. Develop more realistic expectations.

Third, *resolve your anger through problem solving and negotiation.* Janice will have to break free of the ritual of doing things as she's always done them. She must be willing to accept changes in her capabilities, *at this time,* and adjust accordingly. Can she make changes in her work environment which will help her work more efficiently? Can she improve other skills to compensate for the increased time required to perform what were once easily completed tasks? Becoming more efficient and better organized and setting priorities will help Janice make it through her workday. Honest and open communication with her co-workers and employer will ease bad feelings. Being open to change and learning to adapt to her new physical limitations are the answers to Janice's dilemma.

How can Margaret get her family to understand the torment she is going through? Just expecting them to understand is unreasonable, particularly with all of the mixed messages she's sending to her family. She must talk candidly to them. She must learn ways to let them know her feelings before the anger and resentment build up and complicate what is already a difficult situation. Thoughtful communication—letting her family know how to help her—will settle Margaret's problem.

Ken must work around the obstacles that make him feel cheated. Moving forward through these problems will increase his feelings of strength and competence. Triumph over adversity will help eliminate his feelings of being victimized by RA. He must aim to overcome the inequities of having RA by using his energies to seek improvement. But most importantly, he must understand the indiscriminate nature of RA. Nothing he did or did not do caused his condition, and to view it as some form of punishment merely compounds the problem.

Finally, *redirect negative energy by modifying negative thoughts and behaviors.* If it is directed positively, anger can sometimes be useful. Janice, for example, can direct her energies toward finding the *possibilities* instead of clinging to the *impossibilities*. Margaret can trade misdirected anger for her family's help and encouragement. And Ken can exchange resentment for the personal challenge of recovery. They all will feel relieved when they redirect their anger into positive actions.

Depression

Depression is a common feature of RA. People with RA may be envisioning a life filled with pain or feeling old before their time. They may feel cheated. And self-esteem may waver when they find they can't do things they once did with ease. These are good reasons to feel sad, and prolonged or intense sadness can lead to depression.

The following statements contain subtle cues that a person may be depressed:

"I'm too tired to visit the Bensons tonight."
"Nothing's wrong. I just don't have anything to say."
"It's Jimmy's birthday? I forgot."
"I feel okay. I'm just not hungry, that's all."
"I hardly shut my eyes all night."
"Honey, my joints are just too sore tonight."

Feeling melancholy is not the only symptom of depression. Loss of energy, decreased interest in previously enjoyed activities, forgetfulness, loss of appetite or excessive appetite, difficulty sleeping, and decreased libido can all be symptoms of depression. But these same symptoms can be caused by RA, so it's important to clarify their source.

Depression results in further pain, poorer sleep patterns, added muscle tension, and increased fatigue—all of which can lead to deeper depression. This cycle needs to be broken. The primary motivating agent must be *you*, the person with RA.

Managing Depression

Recognizing that you are depressed is very important, but often this alone will not get you out of the doldrums. Depression often falls on people like a heavy veil that seems impossible to lift. It is suffocating, leaving people feeling helpless and vulnerable. If you feel as though you are struggling beneath the weight of depression, you'll need to muster the fortitude that your depression has temporarily concealed. Do whatever it takes to retrieve your personal strengths and rip through the shroud, casting it aside.

Get the facts. What you *think* influences how you *feel*. What are you thinking that might be leading you to feel depressed? Is fact—or imagination—directing you? Are you fearful that you will always suffer this much pain? Or that arthritis will progress until you are eventually wheelchair bound? If so, fiction is dictating your feelings and your depression. You need to become objective enough to respond to facts rather than to unfounded fears. If you can't be objective, consult someone who can, such as your physician.

Get help. There's no question that everyone can benefit from outside help from time to time: *breaking free of depression is a difficult thing to do.* For this reason, anyone who is suffering from depression should feel free to use all available resources. For example, therapists—**psychologists and psychiatrists**—with expertise in chronic conditions can be very helpful to people who are in the process of adjusting to life changes.

Frequently, depression is caused by a chemical imbalance. When this occurs or when the depression is so severe or chronic that the person is having a very hard time coming out of it, a physician may prescribe medications to help lift it.

Talking openly to a good listener sometimes is all that is needed. Friends and loved ones will help you focus on what is important to you and what is worth looking forward to. Talking to people who are having the same experiences that you are having can make you feel less alone (the local chapter of the Arthritis Foundation can put you in touch with a support group in your area).

It's understandable if you feel that you're just not ready to face friends yet. You may need some time to arrange your thoughts and feelings. If being alone becomes a routine, however, you may want to consider seeking professional advice. Remember, this is a new experience for you, and you don't have to try to be your own expert.

Do not isolate yourself from others. Withdrawing from friends and activities because of depression will only increase your sense of loss and loneliness. At first it may seem easier to isolate yourself, because by doing so you can avoid questions, unwanted advice, and assorted comments from others. You may even convince yourself that it is your arthritis that is holding you back. You may be picturing yourself as a wet blanket— a person who is no longer any fun to be with—and make excuses to friends. These friends may begin to feel as if you don't want to see them. Be as honest with them about your feelings as you want to be, but don't avoid your friends. You will still enjoy their company and they, yours. Good friends are good medicine, and enjoying friendship combats depression.

Pursue something you enjoy doing. Think of activities that have lifted your spirits in the past. Getting involved in something that you once had fun doing is a good way to remind yourself of who you are, and enjoying an activity is a good way to ease your mind of other troubles and relieve stress. Write down twenty things that you enjoyed doing in the past, and then try doing some of them.

Focus on today. Learning and practicing stress reduction and relaxation techniques that focus on the mindfulness of the present rather than regrets of the past or worries of the future may also be a tremendous help.

Focus on a positive attitude. Objectively stand back and listen to each negative thought as though someone else were expressing it. Allow yourself to get annoyed at the negative thoughts, and then modify them into something positive. Sometimes focusing on a positive attitude can turn a half-step backward into two steps forward.

Improve self-esteem. Many people feel depressed about their physical appearance or changes in their capabilities. Keep in mind that not all of these changes need be negative. Appropriate exercise, often with new sports such as swimming, will improve your physical condition. Learning new skills, making new acquaintances, learning a new hobby, or attaining new goals will remind you that you are still a bright, innovative person, capable of growth and change. Do what it takes to remain a productive and fulfilled person whose self-esteem continues to grow and improve.

Help others. There is nothing more rewarding than helping another person. Focusing on someone else's problems can help you forget yours. When you view your life through their eyes you will see that you have much to offer other people.

Exercise. Doing exercises as prescribed is an excellent way to relieve your mind of negative thoughts. People often feel better with regular exercise. Athletes have known this for a long time—they actually feel depressed when they don't exercise routinely. This is because exercise helps your body produce endorphins—natural body chemicals that boost your spirits. Don't leave exercise to chance: incorporate it into your routine.

Anxiety, Fear, and Stress

Anxiety. This is a general, sometimes vague, sense of unease or worry. It is generally not directed toward any one issue. Fear, on the other hand, has a definite direction. In RA, fear is usually directed toward immediate and future problems such as pain and the possibility of disability, job loss, medication toxicities, loss of friends, and inability to meet financial obligations. Whenever anxiety and fear overwhelm our ability to cope, stress is the inevitable result.

Fear. What are you afraid of, and what is the basis of your fear? Fear of future adverse consequences associated with RA or its required medications is understandable. But do you assume that every possible complication or toxic reaction will happen to you? That situation is extremely unlikely. This form of worrying drains your energy and slows your progress.

Combat fear with facts. Learn to recognize the early signs of problems; then, if they do occur, you and your physician can act promptly and decisively to counteract them. If you follow this advice you will feel better prepared and less frightened. Confronting each problem as it presents itself will make you feel stronger and better equipped to deal with any future difficulties. Being adequately informed about RA and its course of treatment can be extremely reassuring.

Stress. Stress is a universal aspect of life—a predictable reaction to life's surprises. Our world is constantly changing and presenting us with new situations and environments, and we draw on our resources to make adjustments to these changes. If the magnitude of the changes overwhelms our ability to adjust, we experience stress.

In our daily *routines*, we are aware of potential demands and know how to approach them, but when that routine is altered—when change occurs—we may stumble. Stress associated with change is generally a result of our anxiety and fear of the unknown: we don't know what the future holds, and we may be afraid that we don't have what it takes to meet this unexpected challenge.

Since RA is a life change that has a great deal of unpredictability associated with it, stress is a normal response to it. In fact, the most stressful part of RA is its unpredictability. People with RA do not know what they need to prepare for. The course of the condition varies among individuals and varies over time in the same person. This results in having to make frequent adjustments, which in itself can be stressful. People with RA often say that if they only knew what to expect they might not feel so anxious, they might adjust more easily. If you dwell on potential or unexpected future consequences, such as medication toxicity, medical bills, or pain, you will almost always begin to feel afraid. And, as we have seen, anxiety and fear lead to stress.

Stress changes the pain threshold by opening the pain gate (Chapter 6). Stress also causes physical and mental fatigue, which interferes with restful sleep, further increasing pain. And stress affects the body in other ways; it can result in increased heart rate and perspiration and in elevated blood pressure.

But stress is not always harmful. Stress occurs with positive changes as well as negative ones. Consider how you felt when you graduated from school, bought a house, got married, or went on a long-anticipated vacation. We all know, too, that feeling a little stress can motivate us to get tasks accomplished. Everyone has experienced short-lived deadline pressure and responded to it with increased adrenaline and increased activity. When stress becomes a permanent part of your life, however, it can take its toll on you and your physical health.

You can use coping skills to approach negative stress. First, you must identify the source of stress (*define the problem*). This includes identifying situations that cause you stress at work and at home. Determine which of these can be modified and which cannot. Avoid the frustration of trying to change the unchangeable, and start with a set of goals that can be accomplished.

To solve a stress-related dilemma (*problem solving*), begin by appraising the situation. What are its demands? Are they reasonable at this particular time? If necessary, modify as many of the demands as possible so that they are reasonable for you at this time. Then call on the following problem-solving tactics:

· Propose a reasonable long-term goal (reasonable expectations).
· Plan ahead (include short-term, attainable goals).
· Provide a supportive environment (communication).

· Promote your identified strengths (use all resources).
· Put priorities into perspective (does it need to be done now?).
· Prepare (get organized).
· Place time slots in your schedule to allow for inevitable interruptions and rest breaks (expect the unexpected).
· Pace yourself (one step at a time).
· Positively reappraise the situation and your abilities (modify negative thoughts and behaviors).
· Prove to yourself that you can do it.
· Praise yourself for a job well done.

You can see almost any situation through by calling upon your imagination, and each time you overcome a stressful situation successfully you increase your ability to cope with stress. Each such experience will empower you! Remember, "A great part of courage is having done the thing before" (Ralph Waldo Emerson).

Relieving Tension: Dealing with Anxiety, Fear, and Stress

There are numerous techniques you can use to minimize anxiety, fear, and stress, ranging from the simple to the exotic. It's worth mentioning here that it is often difficult to separate emotional tension from muscle or physical tension. We know that decreasing tension in one area often relieves tension in the other area, so, as you'll see, many of these tactics for relieving emotional tension involve physical activities.

Simple tactics include taking short breaks during your workday to relax, away from the noise and bustle of the workplace. While you relax, collect yourself and redirect the energies that are being drained by stress. At home, a long bath combined with relaxing music can ease your mind and body of tension. Making a detour to the whirlpool or sauna on your way home from work is a good way to wind down from an exhausting day. Gentle muscle massage administered by a friend, spouse, or professional massage therapist can relax tired, tense muscles and decrease your level of stress.

Often, just relaxing your mind by engaging in an enjoyable task or talking with a friend can reduce emotional and physical tension. Taking slow, deep, and regular breaths (preferably from the diaphragm rather than the chest) is another simple but effective way to decrease muscle tension and stress.

One of the more exotic techniques is a deep muscle relaxation technique called **progressive relaxation.** Many people incorporate this technique into their daily and nighttime routines. Begin by finding a quiet place and getting into a comfortable position. Close your eyes. Strongly tense up (clench) your toe muscles for about five seconds. Then relax them, feeling the difference between tension and relaxation. Proceed by alternately tensing and relaxing all of the major muscle groups in your body, from toes to head. When done correctly (doing so takes practice) this technique will leave your body loose and relaxed. Dr. Edmund Jacobson, who first described this technique in 1929, has discovered that it is physically impossible to feel nervous or anxious in any part of our body if our muscles are completely relaxed. This suggests that if we are able to relax the muscles successfully other features of anxiety will be eliminated.

Some individuals incorporate **imagery** into their relaxation techniques. Closing your eyes and imagining yourself in a pleasant, restful place may help you achieve a peaceful state.

Some people have found **biofeedback** to be helpful in controlling chronic tension and pain. This technique involves measuring involuntary body functions such as heart rate, blood pressure, skin temperature, and muscle tension with monitoring equipment that is painlessly attached to the skin. Information about the physical (biological) changes taking place in the body is directly *fed back* to the subject from the equipment. The person being monitored can use this feedback to identify behaviors that bring about pain or tension and can then modify thoughts that induce these changes. The ultimate goal of biofeedback is to achieve mental mastery of the body's responses.

Recognizing that the mind and the body are intimately connected opens other avenues to reduce mental as well as physical tension. Many mind-body therapies follow spiritual traditions of the East. **Meditation** is a fundamental element of many Indian and Chinese practices. A person can develop powers of concentration directed at calming the mind and thus the body.

There are several types of meditation. Most commonly, during meditation, one focuses on a single thing: a word, sound, thought, image or other object. Many choose the breath as their object. It takes a lot of practice to disregard thoughts and push out the "clutter" that occupies valuable space in our mind. This form of meditation is called "concentration meditation." With practice and continued discipline, focusing thoughts becomes easier, and deep states of calmness can be achieved.

A second technique, called "mindfulness" or "insight" meditation, is completely different. It encourages you to attend to the present moment. When thoughts or emotions enter your mind, you observe them without judgment or analysis. You let the thoughts flow freely. As you witness your own thoughts, you bring clarity to what is really on your mind, without defensiveness, intellectualizing, or reaction. This nonjudgmental awareness of your own thoughts and emotions can help bring acceptance and insight. With this clarity of presence, you are free to take the next step. Different techniques work for different people. The important point is that you must *make the time* in your schedule to give any technique a fair trial. How many of us have verbalized at one time or another that we "just need time to think"? Perhaps we should listen to what we are telling ourselves. Meditation, as well as imagery and biofeedback, can affect the way pain and tension are perceived, and can possibly even affect the course of your arthritis.

For many people, prayer and expanded spirituality can provide a sense of order in the face of life's countless challenges. The belief in a greater power helps us to focus on truly significant aspects of our daily lives. Studies have shown that many people are strongly influenced by activities such as prayer and worship. People who participate in these healing activities appear to recover faster from surgery, have reduced pain, and suffer less from stress. How each person broadens his or her spiritual self is an individual expedition with an evolving destination. Bon voyage!

People who are feeling anxious or afraid or who feel that their life or condition is controlling them can use any of these techniques to help. We also speak more about the mind-body connection and its role in healing in Chapter 18, where we review complementary therapies. The important message is that using tactics that sift our extraneous sources of stress will allow you to relax your mind and body so you can focus on what is really important for you and your loved ones.

Dealing with Friends and Family

Your loved ones need to progress through these emotional changes with you. You will want their help and empathy, for example (but not their pity). You will probably want them to acknowledge your limitations without viewing them as weaknesses. You will need the support of your loved ones, but you won't want them to hover or be oversolicitous.

From their perspective, your loved ones are also struggling with the changes that your having RA has introduced. They may be uncertain about how to approach you. Should they offer their help? Should they allow you to do what you can? Should they pretend that nothing's changed? They will need your guidance. You must set the tone and direction for your future interactions. Your messages to others should be clear and concise. You must communicate with them and not expect them to understand simply because they love you. Mixed messages result in misunderstandings and hurt feelings.

Asking for Help

It is difficult to ask for help with tasks that you once were able to do on your own, but you will need to do this from time to time. If you learn to ask for help in a way that lets you keep your sense of independence and confidence, you will be much more likely to ask for the help you need. And when you get needed help, your feelings of frustration or anger can be avoided. Learn to ask clearly and without ambiguity, so that the person you're asking knows exactly how you need to be helped. Consider the following unproductive approaches:

"I'll just do it myself." (Martyrdom is overvalued.)

"Can't you see I'm in pain and can't do this?" (It does no good to try to induce guilt in someone else.)

"Wash the dishes or *else*." (People who feel as if they are being punished for your arthritis will sooner or later come to resent your requests for assistance.)

"I *can* do it, but I think it's about time for you to do something around here." (Denial has the potential to develop into antagonism.)

Now consider the following requests, messages that preserve self-esteem while constructively conveying the need for assistance:

"Here's what I need help with. I know I can count on you." (Describe the task and show appreciation; the response will almost certainly be positive.)

"I'm certain I can do this part alone, but I could really use your help with the rest of it." (Be specific about your needs, including what you *don't* need help with.)

"I'll clean up the living room if you'll vacuum the rug." (Negotiation allows equal input from everyone.)

Remember, your attitude has a far greater effect on your personal interactions than your disabilities do.

The Special Case of Children

A parent who has RA may find the adventure of childrearing especially challenging. For one thing, children require structure and routine, and it's hard to maintain consistency when you have a condition that fluctuates. On good days you may not need help from your kids, or you may be able to participate in activities with them. On bad days you may require their help and understanding. Despite the unpredictable nature of your arthritis, you must try to be consistent in your interactions with your children and your response to them.

For example, if one week you say, "Jimmy, I want you to clean up your room. I don't feel well," and a week later, when you're feeling better, you say "Jimmy, why don't you go watch cartoons while I clean up your room?" it's not going to take too long for Jimmy to realize that he will have to do more when you are feeling bad and will be rewarded when you feel well. It's far better to separate Jimmy's responsibilities from your physical condition: "Jimmy, you're six years old now, and we think you're big enough to pick up your room."

Erase from your mind any feelings of guilt you may have for not doing everything for your children. Guilt provides no positive direction and only allows your children to manipulate you. Redirect your energy toward teaching lessons in responsibility and independence which will last your children a lifetime. A final note: there's nothing to prevent you from rewarding children for taking on new responsibilities. This is another real-life lesson, because we frequently are rewarded for a job well done.

A second caution to parents is to avoid making a promise such as "We'll do this if I feel well." When something's coming up which is important to the child, develop a backup plan. This may entail something as simple as making it okay for the other parent and the child to participate in the activity without you. If you are a single parent, think about asking the parents of your child's friends to help out if you are feeling ill. *Do not wait until the day of the occasion* to make alternate plans, as this may leave you feeling trapped. Again, the goal is not to link your child's hopes too closely to your level of health on a given day.

Love and Intimacy

At some time nearly everyone's love life is affected by the daily stresses of living. Changes in energy, emotions, personal body image, and self-esteem directly affect how you feel as a sexual person. If you do not feel attractive, for example, you will not expect others to be attracted to you. To improve or renew your intimate relationships, you must first address the issues of energy, emotions, body image, and self-esteem in your life. When you start feeling strong and in control of your life, everything will change for you. With renewed confidence and self-esteem you will realize that you are a loving (and lovable) person capable of, and deserving of, an enduring and fulfilling relationship with your partner.

One key to a successful, loving relationship is communication, and this is particularly true when one partner has a health problem. It is not always easy for people to discuss their intimate concerns, however. But consider the following questions. If they are left unasked—and unanswered—they can seriously damage a relationship.

· Am I still attractive to my partner?
· Am I hurting her?
· Is he still interested?
· Why isn't he more concerned with my needs?

Misunderstandings over issues of intimacy can linger for months if they are not addressed. As a result, one or both partners may begin to avoid intimacy and even situations that may lead to intimacy. Once this pattern of aloofness is begun, it may be difficult to break. *Communication is the key.* Express your concerns to your partner:

· Do you still find me attractive?
· Am I hurting you?
· I want to make love but you seem distant. What's going on?
· Maybe you don't realize that sex first thing in the morning is often painful for me. Can we schedule a rendezvous for lunchtime?

Dr. Jackson Rainer of Webb University (Enliven, 2000) believes that intimacy issues are often ignored. He recommends working toward *intimacy* rather than placing too much emphasis on intercourse. He believes that "the biggest sex organ is the skin, and the best sex organ is the brain." Couples should focus on "closeness, touch, pleasure, and contact" rather than the act of sex. He also gives the following approaches:

· Talk about intimacy issues in a setting away from the bedroom.
· Be straightforward and concrete in your communication.
· Take small steps, and keep the dialogue going.
· Begin to court and date each other again.

People are appropriately becoming more comfortable talking with their doctors about problems with sexual function. Pain, fatigue, and medications can have an impact on libido as well as other sexual activities. In some men with RA, erectile dysfunction has been reported. If this is the case, we strongly encourage an evaluation by your physician. Low androgen (male hormone) levels have been discovered in some men with RA. Therapy with testosterone in those individuals may make a difference in sexual function. Testosterone replacement has been shown to have other positive effects in men with RA and low androgen levels (Cutolo, 2000). Women can also be affected with sexual difficulties. Issues regarding body image and anxieties regarding health have been shown to affect many women and their sexuality (Gutweniger et al., 1999). Please do not ignore these issues. Help is available to work through these complicated concerns, but you need to ask.

As suggested earlier in this book, there may be times during which physical limitations—fatigue, painful joints, and restricted motion—interfere with your sex life. Creativity is *very* helpful in overcoming these obstacles. Upon request, the Arthritis Foundation will send you a free pamphlet called "Guide to Intimacy and Arthritis," which provides guidelines for comfortable physical intimacy. Here are some suggestions:

· Plan for sex at the time of day when you feel best.
· Take pain relief medicine ahead of time so that it takes effect before intercourse.
· Pace activities during the day to avoid becoming fatigued before sex.
· Perform range-of-motion exercises to relax your joints before sex.
· Take a warm bath or shower before sex to relax both you and your joints.

Planning for sexual activity may seem awkward and contrived when you first start doing it. But it need not be. With creativity and imagination the preparation can become an exciting and stimulating addition to your relationship. It also sends a message to your partner that you desire to continue and expand your intimate relationship.

Friends and Relatives

Friends and relatives can be a wonderful source of support and inspiration for you. Some of them will show great sensitivity and understanding and will help you through trying times almost instinctively. Other people—most people, in fact—will look to you for direction. You must let them know that you value their friendship and company, and you must show them how they can support you when times are hard. If you must decline a social invitation because of your arthritis, be sure to let people know that you want to be included in future get-togethers.

Friends and relatives can also be a tremendous source of irritation. Remember, there are many, many people who do not know much about RA. Although most people mean well, they may say the wrong thing. Our recommendation is to use private humor as a way to cope with the dumb comment or the thoughtless statement. So, when someone makes an inappropriate remark, think about how you *wish you could* respond . . . then wait a few seconds . . . and instead make a constructive response to your friend or relative. Here are some ideas:

The *should have* comment: "You *should have* exercised more; then you wouldn't have arthritis."
Think: "You *should have* gone to charm school."
Say: "That's an interesting hypothesis. Although exercise is important, its absence hasn't been shown to be linked to the development of rheumatoid arthritis."

The *should* comment: "You *should* drink six pints of apricot juice each day to cure your arthritis."

Think: "You *should* learn that silence can be golden."
Say: "A balanced diet is very important for all people, including those with rheumatoid arthritis."

The *could have* comment: "You should feel lucky, you *could have* developed cancer."
Think: "I do feel lucky, you *could have* been someone whose opinion mattered to me."
Say: "I do feel good that I have a condition I can cope with successfully."

The *I've got a relative with arthritis* comment: "My third cousin twice removed has that kind of arthritis and she's crippled."
Think: "I wish you were twice removed from me."
Say: "Did you know that there are more than one hundred types of arthritis? With early treatment and therapy, few people with arthritis today develop serious handicaps."

The brilliant observer: "Did you know that your hands are swollen?"
Think: "Thank you for the brilliant observation, Einstein."
Say: "Yes, I did. Thank you for your concern."

The doting relative: "Serve your sister her dinner! Can't you see she has arthritis?"
Think: "Would you mind chewing and swallowing it for me, too?"
Say: "Mom, I appreciate your concern, but I would really like to do the things I can do alone. There will be things I'll need assistance with in the future, and I'm glad that I can count on all of you for your help."

Get the idea? You'll probably be surprised at the type of comment that will pop into your head in these circumstances. Thinking silently of a humorous response is a good way to ventilate your annoyance without alienating the person who makes a thoughtless comment. Remember, most people are trying to be supportive. Be patient and direct them in their efforts. Do not get angry or hurt. Use your energy to educate them about RA so that they won't continue making senseless comments.

For More Information

Two helpful pamphlets, "A Guide to Intimacy with Arthritis" and "Managing Your Stress," are available from the Arthritis Foundation (1330 W. Peachtree St., Atlanta, Ga. 30309; 1-800-283-7800).

PART III

Exercise
and
Rehabilitation

•

CHAPTER 8

Protecting Your Joints

•

Inflamed joints are more easily injured than joints that are not inflamed. Everyone who has rheumatoid arthritis (RA) must learn how to *protect* his or her joints, giving special attention to the joints in the hands and wrists, since these are particularly vulnerable to injury during daily activity.

Joint protection involves more than a list of things to do and not to do; it is a philosophy that should be incorporated into one's daily routine. At first the strategies may seem awkward or inefficient, and having to stop and think about how you move before you move can seem bothersome. With practice, however, these tactics will become routine. Joint protection will become second nature to you.

After your arthritis has improved, you should continue to follow the principles of joint protection. Your reward will be decreased pain and stiffness as well as preservation of the best possible joint function.

In this chapter each of the principles of joint protection is discussed along with examples of how these guidelines may be used. We recommend that you incorporate these guidelines into your daily life. An **occupational therapist** can help you understand these principles and help you apply them to your particular situation. Ask your physician to refer you to an occupational therapist, especially if you're having difficulty putting these principles into practice.

Joint Protection Guidelines

Respect your pain. Increased pain is a warning that you are overtaxing your joints. You should heed this warning and modify the activity. This principle is discussed in detail in Chapter 6; we mention it again here because it is so very important.

Balance rest with activity. Organizing your schedule so that you alternate energy-intensive activities with more restful ones will stretch your energy reserves and protect your joints as well. Conserving your energy by avoid-ing unnecessary tasks will leave you with more energy to exercise and do the necessary ones.

Maintain your muscle strength. Strong muscles provide additional sup-port to your joints and help protect them from undue stress. (Chapters 9 and 10 describe ways to build and maintain muscle strength.)

Avoid activities that cannot be stopped. Try to steer clear of prolonged activities that leave you no room or opportunity to rest. Consider that standing in a long line without being able to sit down will leave you fa-tigued. With some planning you can avoid peak hours and long lines at the post office, bank, and grocery store. Carrying a package for a long dis-tance—across a parking lot, for example—is another activity that can wear you out. Again, the best way to avoid this is to plan ahead: keep a portable or fold-up cart in your car. This will allow you to transport the object without exerting much energy and to take small rest breaks during the trek if you need to.

Avoid positions that promote deformity. Sometimes ligaments and mus-cles become stretched with the inflammation of arthritis. This may result in unequal forces being exerted across the joints, creating a situation in which the joints *drift,* or change their alignment. This is known as joint deformity. The word *deformity* is frightening for most people. The use of the word within this setting, however, merely describes a change in the normal positioning (and, sometimes, function) of joints. Later in this chapter we will describe positions that make deformity worse; these po-sitions are to be avoided.

Utilize the largest joint and the strongest muscle available to complete a task. It makes good sense to call upon your most powerful joints and muscles to perform any given task. In this way you avoid putting stress upon smaller, less powerful joints and muscles. Consider the task of lift-ing a heavy book. If you pick the book up between your thumb and fin-gers, the fingers and wrist will have a great deal of stress placed on them. Instead, if you pick the book up by sliding your hands underneath the book, palms up, and then lifting it, your arm muscles and elbows will do the work, and you'll avoid putting extra stress on your wrists and fingers.

Avoid remaining in one position or using muscles in one stationary posi-tion for long periods of time. Remaining in one position for too long pro-motes stiffness or a **gelling** effect on inflamed joints. Muscles also become fatigued when you use them from a stationary position for long periods.

(Think about how your muscles begin to cramp when you write for lengthy periods without stopping or readjusting the pencil or pen.) Stiffness of joints and muscles can be avoided by changing to a different position every fifteen to twenty minutes. Frequent stretching also helps prevent joints from losing range of motion. Again, take frequent breaks, stretch, and change positions before muscle fatigue sets in.

Utilize splinting as needed. A splint is a fabricated support that is designed to stabilize inflamed joints. In RA, a splint has three basic functions. It can be designed to (1) rest an inflamed joint by partially or completely immobilizing it, (2) protect a weakened joint from injury by supporting it, and (3) improve function of a damaged joint.

Splints should only be used if they decrease pain and inflammation or improve function. There is no good evidence available that splints prevent deformity. On the other hand, it has been proven that incorrect or prolonged use of splints can lead to increased stiffness, decreased strength, and decreased motion. If you believe that you are receiving no benefit from a prescribed splint, discuss this with your physician or occupational therapist.

Utilize assistive equipment as needed. There are numerous catalogues listing accessories that are useful for people who have arthritis—so many, in fact, that the choices may be overwhelming. Our advice is to use as little in the way of assistive equipment as possible, because these devices can actually *interfere* with your ability to function independently if you rely on them too heavily or if you use too many of them. This is not to say that there aren't many situations in which a specific item can help you considerably and spare your joints from excessive stress. The Arthritis Foundation produces an excellent resource called *Tips for Good Living with Arthritis*. This book will help you select and obtain useful self-help equipment.

Protecting Specific Joints

The following hints for protecting specific joints have proven to be quite effective. Please note that you needn't observe these principles for joints in which you have no arthritis involvement.

Hands and Wrists

Finger and wrist joints tend to slowly drift out of their natural alignment as the result of chronic inflammation, as illustrated in Figures 9, 10, and 11. To avoid contributing to these deformities adhere to these principles.

Figure 9. Wrist-deforming forces

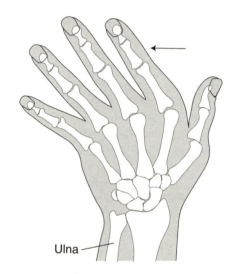

Ulna

Figure 10. Ulnar drift

· When stirring foods, hold the utensil with your thumb on top (as if you were stabbing a block of ice with an ice pick) and stir with shoulder motion.
· Avoid hanging a purse strap over your wrist or carrying heavy suitcases.
· Avoid supporting your body weight on your wrists and hands. For example, do not lean on your hands while standing against a table edge.
· Avoid stressful wringing and twisting motions. (Use an electric rather than a manual can opener. Roll hand-washed items in a towel.)
· Do not wring your washcloth out, let the cloth drip dry.
· Do not grip items tightly or hold onto them for long periods. Too tight a grip increases deforming pressures.
· Modify the size of articles that you grasp daily. You can enlarge the grips on pencils, pens, toothbrushes, and other utensils by placing the handles inside a foam hair curler or wrapping them with soft foam rubber.

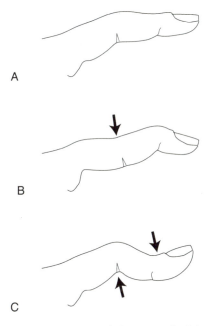

A

B

C

Figure 11. Finger joints: *A*, normal; *B*, swan neck; *C*, boutonnière

· Avoid actions that push your other fingers toward your little finger (Figure 10). To dial on a rotary dial telephone, use an unsharpened pencil, holding it with your thumb on the top. When reading, don't hold a book in a way that puts weight on your fingers (use a bookholder). Don't rest your chin on top of your fingers. Lift and carry objects with palms, not with your fingers. When getting up from a chair, use your palms rather than your fingers to push off.
· Open jars by putting pressure on the top with your palm and twisting from the shoulder rather than by gripping the lid with your fingers.

Remember to use the largest joint and the strongest muscle available to complete the job. For example, shut doors with your hip or upper arm rather than your fingers.

Splints. The splints that are available today are made of lighter weight materials and are smaller than they were in the past. They are also more comfortable and attractive than splints used to be. The ring splint illustrated in Figure 12 is an example of a modern splint that can be used by persons with swan neck (Figure 11B) or boutonnière (Figure 11C) deformity, if the splint improves function.

Figure 12. Ring splint

Figure 13. Functional wrist splint

Figure 14. Resting hand splint

Hand and wrist splints can be either commercially fabricated (purchased over the counter) or custom fit by an occupational therapist or orthotist. (An **orthotist** is an expert in the development and application of splints, braces, and other supports to improve function or decrease pain and inflammation.) The functional wrist splint illustrated in Figure 13 is useful because it allows some movement at the fingers while immobilizing the wrist. Some physicians prescribe a resting hand splint (Figure 14) to be worn at night to rest finger and wrist joints. Remember, splints should only be used if they relieve pain or improve function.

Assistive equipment. People with hand and wrist problems may find use of the following equipment helpful:

· built-up handles
· faucet turners or levers
· key adaptors or levers
· button hook
· elastic shoelaces
· door opener
· car door opener or lever
· loop scissors
· luggage carrier
· mitt potholder
· padded wrist rest for computer keyboard or typewriter
· battery-powered or electric toothbrush

Elbows and Shoulders

A position that can cause deformity in the elbow is illustrated in Figure 15A, in which the inappropriate use of a cane is shown putting stress on the elbow joint. Figure 15B illustrates a walking device that does not put this stress on the elbow and which cuts down on stress to the wrists, as well.

Here, as with hands and wrists, the principle is to avoid putting stress on the joint in a way that contributes to deformity. For example, when you are carrying heavy objects, keep them as close to your body as possible so that your spine can relieve some of the stress on your shoulders, elbows, and wrists.

Assistive equipment. Assistive equipment to relieve stress on shoulders and elbows includes items that have extended handles and items that allow you to carry things without using your arms.

· extended handles on combs, hairbrushes, toothbrushes, utensils
· extended handle dustpan
· elbow crutch
· over-the-shoulder pouch
· knapsack
· small cart for carrying items (a folding shopping cart, for example)

Figure 15. *A,* elbow-deforming forces; *B,* forearm cane

Hips and Knees

People whose hips and knees are affected by arthritis need to make every effort to keep their weight down. This will limit the amount of pressure that is put on these joints.

One technique for avoiding putting undue pressure on hips and knees is to use your whole body to rise from a sitting position. Slide forward as far as you can in the seat and then lean forward over your knees and swing up. Try to push off with your forearms or palms (avoid using your fingers). Elevating yourself in the chair with a pillow will help.

Assistive equipment. People with arthritis in the hips and knees may find the following equipment helpful. Remember that these assistive devices should not be *overused*. Reaching, for example, is good exercise, and if reaching is not painful for you, you probably are better off *not* using a long-handled reacher.

· elevated seat with arm rests
· raised toilet seat
· stool
· shower bench
· extended shoehorn
· long-handled reacher
· tub grab bars
· walking aids (cane, walker)

Ankles and Feet

RA in the feet can cause swelling and stretched ligaments, and over time the foot often becomes broader and the toes higher than they were before. One of the best ways to protect your feet and ankles is to wear the proper footwear, because a shoe that fits poorly can injure sensitive toes and feet and cause further deformity.

Do not under any circumstances purchase a shoe that rubs or causes pressure and then expect to break it in. This will only come to pass at the expense of your feet. The best advice really is, "If the shoe fits, wear it." When shopping for shoes, look for the following features:

· light weight
· deep enough toe box to clear top of toes; deeper if insert is needed
· wide enough not to pinch toes together
· breathable, supple uppers (leather or canvas); seamless deerskin or calfskin are the best materials
· one inch or lower heel
· good shock absorption when heel contacts ground; crepe soles are excellent for this
· good support along the inside of the foot
· durable, stiff back for support

People with RA often have difficulty finding shoes that are comfortable, practical, and stylish. If the arthritis in your feet is mild, shoes that are deep and wide, such as good supportive walking shoes or athletic shoes, will usually suffice.

If you have minor deformities of the feet, you may require an insert, or orthosis, for your shoes. These foot supports can be purchased over the counter, or they can be specially designed for your feet by a **podiatrist, orthotist,** or **pedorthist.** Supports are designed to relieve pressure on sensitive areas by distributing the pressure to other areas of the foot. Some orthoses can actually prevent or even correct deformity. You will need to purchase shoes that are wide and deep enough to accommodate the orthosis. Many shoe stores sell special shoes for this purpose. Call ahead and ask if the store carries extra wide, extra deep shoes.

Sometimes an extra piece of rubber or leather (*metatarsal bar*) is applied externally to the sole. This takes pressure off the ball of the foot, frequently an area of discomfort.

If you have severe foot damage or deformity you may require specially made shoes. Orthopedic shoes or custom-made shoes can be fabricated from a cast of your feet. Some newer versions are more stylish than the classic orthopedic shoe. Your doctor, therapist, orthopedic surgeon, or podiatrist may be able to give you the name of the best manufacturer of orthopedic shoes in your area. These shoes are generally quite expensive, so ask around before you invest your money. It is important that you select a provider who is willing to make adjustments if the first pair feels uncomfortable to you. Also, find out whether a second pair can be purchased at a reduced fee.

Splints are occasionally recommended for the back of the foot and the ankle. Your physician will tell you whether a foot splint might be useful for you.

Finally, here is some excellent advice from Dr. John Ward and Dr. Carolee Moncur of the University of Utah Medical Center about foot care for people with arthritis:

· Keep your feet meticulously clean and dry, particularly between your toes.
· Examine your feet often for signs of stress.
· Look for blisters and pressure sores. Change your shoes or get professional advice if these signs of stress develop.
· Avoid chemical agents or cutting to remove calluses; they have formed for a reason. Find out what that reason is.
· Cut your toenails straight across.
· Plan ahead to avoid excessive walking when your feet are painful.
· Keep your weight low.

For More Information

The Arthritis Foundation's Tips for Good Living with Arthritis (2001) has hundreds of joint protection tips as well as lists of resources. Order from a bookstore or from the Arthritis Foundation, 1330 W. Peachtree St., Atlanta, Ga. 30309; 1-800-207-8633.

Useful catalogs are available from the following sources:

Aids for Arthritis, Inc., 35 Wakefield Drive, Medford, N.J. 08055; 1-800-654-0707; *www.aidsforarthritis.com.*

Ergonomic Solutions, 129 N. Sylvan Drive, Mundelein, Ill. 60060-4949; 1-800-755-4950; *www.goergo.com.*

Ergo Source, P.O. Box 695, Wayzata, Minn. 55391; 1-800-969-4374.

North Coast Medical Consumer Products Division, 18305 Sutter Blvd., Morgan Hill, Calif. 95037; 1-800-235-7054.

Sammons Preston Storefront (enrichment catalogue), 1-800-323-5547.

Sears Home HealthCare, 3737 Grader St., Suite 110, Garland, Tex. 75041; 1-800-326-1750.

Smith and Nephew, P.O. Box 1005, Germantown, Wisc. 53022; 1-800-558-8633.

CHAPTER 9

Exercise and Rheumatoid Arthritis

•

Should you exercise or should you rest? In this book we have advised you to do both, which at first must seem contradictory. In truth, though, both appropriate exercise *and* adequate rest are important in the treatment of rheumatoid arthritis (RA).

Appropriate exercise can only be managed through an *individualized* rehabilitation program, one that contains the right balance of exercise and rest *for you*. Devising such a program, of course, requires some knowledge of how RA is affecting *you*.

It wasn't so long ago that generalizations were made about patients with RA without regard for their degree of arthritis—but no longer. Now we know that a program that doesn't take the individual's needs into account is destined to be unsafe or unproductive, or both.

Trends in Therapeutic Advice

Proper treatment for RA, including the benefits of exercise, has been the subject of debate for decades. Understanding the historical change in attitude about exercise may help you understand the thinking behind what your physician or therapist is telling you now.

In the 1950s and 1960s, people with RA were routinely treated with bed rest. It was not uncommon, in fact, for a person with RA to be placed in the hospital for one or two months in an attempt to bring the arthritis under control. Since inflamed joints do improve with bed rest (when inflamed joints are splinted or immobilized, the swelling, pain, and heat decrease), the practice continued. In this same time period, exercises were rarely prescribed for *any* arthritis patient (regardless of how well controlled the arthritis was) for fear that the person's condition would worsen.

In time, some health care providers questioned the logic behind prolonged bed rest, which exerts negative effects on the body: muscles weaken, bones lose calcium and become more brittle, and overall fitness diminishes. Although joint inflammation improves with bed rest, people get out of shape while their arthritis is getting under control.

Gradually, health care providers began prescribing exercises for their patients, and over time the amount of prescribed exercise has increased. Gentle range-of-motion exercises, aimed at preserving joint motion, and cautious muscle-strengthening exercises became essential components of the exercise regimen.

In the past twenty years, people have become much more exercise conscious, and trends in therapeutic advice for people with RA reflect this. In the 1970s and 1980s, for example, several inspired investigators decided to see what would happen if they increased the level of exercise in patients whose arthritis was under control. Marion Minor, a registered physical therapist at the University of Missouri-Columbia, as well as other researchers, reported interesting results. They discovered that some individuals with arthritis can perform more advanced strengthening exercises as well as low-impact aerobic exercises with positive effects. These people appeared to benefit from the exercise in numerous ways: they had improved stamina, less fatigue, and better ability to function, and they spent less time away from work and more time away from the hospital.

What physicians and others have learned from changes in treatment adds up to this: You should exercise. Appropriate exercise can improve your energy and strength, increase joint stability, help prevent joint deformities, decrease pain, and allow you to function better. But exercise affects more than just the symptoms of arthritis; it helps build stronger bones, promotes self-esteem, improves the quality of sleep, and decreases muscle tension and anxiety. A fitness program faithfully adhered to will also benefit your lungs, your heart, and your circulation.

The recommended amount and type of exercise depend on the degree of inflammation and the pattern of joint involvement. In this chapter and the next we present a general guide to appropriate exercise and review some precautions as well as some commonly prescribed exercises. It is important to bear in mind that we cannot perform here the skilled evaluation that your physician and physical therapist trained in arthritis can; nor can we give you the individualized advice they can offer. By determining your specific needs, these health care professionals can prescribe an exercise program that will improve *your* function. You need to seek their advice before embarking on an exercise program.

Types of Exercise

Three major forms of exercise are prescribed for people with RA: range of motion, muscle strengthening, and endurance.

Range of Motion

Range of motion refers to the full range of movements that a joint can make. Range-of-motion exercises involve moving each joint as far as it can comfortably be moved in all directions. The goal of this form of exercise is to decrease stiffness and pain, maintain flexibility, and improve the function of the joints. As we have seen, inflammation and decreased use can impair function in the joints, and these exercises are designed to prevent that loss. No weights are used.

Stretching exercises are similar to range-of-motion exercises, but these exercises involve stretching the joint to a limit just beyond that which is comfortable. Joints should never be stretched to the point of excessive pain, however, and they should never be "bounced" in an effort to increase joint motion.

Range-of-motion and stretching exercises are fundamental in the warm-up stage for any exercise program. They should be performed once or twice per day and they can be performed whenever you need to decrease stiffness in the joints.

Strengthening

Strengthening exercises increase your muscle strength and muscle tone, allowing you to function with less muscle fatigue and more joint stability. Thus, muscles that are strengthened through exercise actually help protect the joints. Strengthening exercises are also necessary because muscles that are not used (generally because use causes pain) become smaller (become atrophied), and this causes them to become weaker. Also, tendons and ligaments can stretch and loosen in response to swelling in and around the joints, decreasing joint stability; strengthening exercises can help the joints compensate for these changes caused by RA.

Isometric exercises involve simply tightening, or contracting, muscles (called *muscle setting*), an activity that helps maintain muscle strength. Isometric strengthening exercises involve *maximally* tightening your muscles by pushing or pulling against a fixed object, *without* moving your joints. *Moving your joints in opposition to high resistance should always be avoided.* One example of an isometric strengthening exercise is pushing against a wall without moving your shoulders, elbows, or wrists. With this exercise the arm muscles contract and get stronger but, since the joints are not moving, the joints are protected from increased stress.

Isometric strengthening exercises may also be performed by using *exercise bands*. These are elastic bands (or tubing) that stretch slightly but are very strong. They may be purchased commercially (Thera-Band and Thera-Tube are two name brands), or they may be fabricated from materials you already have in the home (such as an *elastic* belt, bungee cords, rubber tubing, or garden hoses). Adjustable trouser belts that are some-what stretchable work well because you can adjust the size of the loop. You can also double over an elastic belt to decrease the amount of stretch or create a smaller loop. Several examples of isometric exercises using exercise bands are described in the next chapter.

One note of caution: Exercising with weights can stress an inflamed joint. You should avoid this kind of exercise (called *isotonic strengthening exercises*) unless your therapist or doctor instructs you otherwise.

Endurance

Endurance or *aerobic exercises* are designed to increase overall fitness. They prepare your body to perform tasks over a period of time without becoming fatigued or exhausted. They improve your body's efficiency in using oxygen from the blood supply. Circulation, heart function, and respiration (breathing) improve, as well. Endurance exercises compatible with RA include swimming, walking, bicycling, and even some forms of low-impact aerobics, depending on the extent of arthritic involvement of lower extremity joints. Aerobic exercise can also increase muscle strength.

Starting an Exercise Program

An exercise program is made up of three crucial components: warm-up, workout, and cool-down. Most people find that an exercise program occupies about thirty minutes daily, usually ten minutes of warming up, fifteen minutes of working out, and five minutes of cooling down—but this may vary. You should never exercise to the point of extreme fatigue or exhaustion. Start low and go slow, and work your way up! In this way you can make progress without suffering setbacks.

People with RA need to schedule their exercise to coincide with the time of day when they are most rested and have the least pain.

Warm-up

A warm-up is necessary to allow the joints and muscles to loosen up slowly, in preparation for the workout. *Tight joints and muscles should not be exercised.* Warm-up range-of-motion and stretching exercises prepare muscles for more intense exercise.

Workout

The workout that's best for you is determined by the degree of inflammation in your joints. Generally, unless your joints are very inflamed, a workout includes strengthening and aerobic exercises. When joints are very inflamed, the workout may consist only of range-of-motion exercises.

Cool-down

Cool-down relaxes muscles and allows the heart rate and breathing rate to return to their before-workout rate. A cool-down also helps prevent postexercise pain or anxiety. Cool-down exercises can be range-of-motion exercises or aerobic exercises performed in slow motion.

Exercises That Are Right for You

Exercise recommendations vary greatly, depending on the degree of arthritis activity present in the joints. Before undertaking any exercise program, you should always review it with the physician or physical therapist who is most familiar with your specific situation. The key to developing and following an effective rehabilitation and exercise program is to know *your* arthritis.

You may already appreciate that your arthritis can vary greatly over time. You may have experienced a severe flare-up of arthritis in the past after you overexerted yourself. If you know the pattern of your own arthritis, you will be the best judge of which exercises make you feel better and which ones only make you feel worse.

In describing model exercise programs in the rest of this chapter, we have, for the sake of convenience, divided RA into three different levels of activity: very inflamed, moderately inflamed, and controlled. We recognize that this is an artificial division, however, and that few people fit neatly into any one of these categories all the time. Individuals have different exercise needs. We'd like to stress once again that no one with RA should begin an exercise program without obtaining the advice of a health care professional who is familiar with that individual's needs.

For People with Very Inflamed Joints

The very inflamed joint is also known as an *acute joint* or a *highly active joint*. The joint will usually be warm, tender, and swollen. A joint is very inflamed if you experience significant discomfort when you move it through a gentle range-of-motion exercise. There is generally significant morning stiffness in very inflamed joints, as well. You may feel fatigue or muscle discomfort. This is often the level of arthritic activity people mean when they describe their arthritis as *flaring up*.

General exercise program guidelines for people with very inflamed joints include the following:

1. Move each *affected* joint through five repetitions of each range-of-motion exercise once or twice per day.
   Goal: Maintain motion and flexibility in joints.
   Precautions: Do not stretch joints beyond the point at which you feel increased pain. Do not push yourself to extreme fatigue.
2. Tighten each muscle *without moving the joint,* and maintain tension for six seconds once or twice per day.
   Goal: Prevent muscle weakening.
   Precautions: Do not use elastic bands or perform other forms of isometric strengthening at this point. Simply flex and tighten the muscles.

For People with Moderately Inflamed Joints

Moderately inflamed joints are also known as *subacute* joints. Although the inflammation is moderate, these joints still cause some discomfort, and pain increases after the joint has been stressed. For example, you may not notice moderate inflammation in your shoulder until you attempt to retrieve an object from a high shelf. And moving moderately inflamed finger joints might not cause you any discomfort until you try to unscrew the lid of a jar. Subacute joints may have morning stiffness, but it does not last as long as it does in highly active joints.

General exercise program guidelines for people with moderately inflamed joints include the following:

1. Move joints through three, four, or five repetitions of each range-of-motion exercise. Do two or three stretches until you feel that you are at your maximum range of motion, then add one or two more stretches to be sure. Do this once or twice per day.
   Goals: Maintain and slowly increase motion and flexibility. Increase muscle tone.
   Precautions: Cut back the number of repetitions if increased swelling or pain occurs.
2. Incorporate isometric strengthening exercises into your regimen. Hold each contracted muscle against a fixed resistance for six seconds without moving your joints. Elastic bands or other forms of fixed resistance can be used. Use about three-quarters of your maximum strength (or less, if pain occurs). Do this one, two, or three times with each muscle group, taking a ten-second break between each contraction. Isometric strengthening exercises are usually performed only once daily.
   Goal: Increase muscle strength.

Precautions: Your joints should be kept immobile during this form of therapy. Keep the tension in your muscles, not in your joints.

3. Gradual addition of endurance exercises may be appropriate at this stage. Adding a swimming program is often recommended, because the buoyancy of the water relieves stress on joints. Other forms of aerobic exercise may be recommended if your hips, knees, and feet are not inflamed. Before adding exercises such as walking and bicycling to your program, talk it over with your physician.

    Goal: Increase endurance and fitness.

    Precautions: Check with your doctor to see if you are ready for aerobic exercises.

For People with Controlled Joints

The *stable* or *inactive* joint is one which was previously inflamed but is now under satisfactory control. It is not necessarily a normal joint, because damage may have occurred in the past and changed its appearance and function.

Controlled or stable joints are generally not warm to the touch. They also display only minimal morning stiffness and tenderness. They may appear enlarged but are usually not filled with fluid.

Exercise recommendations for controlled joints depend on the amount of damage remaining as a consequence of past inflammation. General guidelines include the following:

1. Continue daily range-of-motion exercises with a maximum of ten repetitions. You can decrease number of repetitions to two or three when maximal range of motion has been attained.

    Goal: Maintain and increase motion and flexibility.

    Precautions: Cut back repetitions if increased pain or swelling becomes evident.

2. Continue isometric strengthening exercises as with moderately inflamed joints. Once maximum strength is achieved you will be able to cut down on these exercises and devote more time to aerobic exercise. Your therapist may also suggest a form of isotonic exercise with small weights, if your joints are under excellent control and do not show any sign of significant damage.

    Goal: Increase strength.

    Precautions: All strengthening exercise programs should be reviewed with your doctor or therapist. Placing inappropriate stress on damaged joints can result in increased deformity. Never use weights without checking first with your doctor or therapist.

3. Endurance exercises are most important in this stage to help you re-

gain aerobic conditioning lost when the arthritis was more active. Swimming is still the best form of exercise, but other forms of low-impact aerobics may be considered (for example, walking, bicycling, low-impact dancing). Half an hour of aerobic exercise three times weekly will increase your fitness. As you grow stronger and spend more time with endurance exercises, you can eliminate some of your strengthening exercises, although it is a good idea to continue range-of-motion exercises with affected joints. This will prevent shrinking or shortening of the muscle.

Goal: Increase endurance and fitness.

Precautions: Review all aerobic exercises with a physician who is familiar with your degree of joint damage and other specific health problems that may interfere with aerobic exercise.

For More Information

A free pamphlet called "Exercise and Your Arthritis," which has helpful tips for more effective exercise, is available from the Arthritis Foundation (1330 W. Peachtree St., Atlanta, Ga. 30309; 1-800-283-7800).

The Missouri Arthritis Rehabilitation Research and Training Center is the only federally funded arthritis rehabilitation research and training center. Excellent resources are available through its Web site (www .muhealth.org/arthritis) or by writing or calling (130 A. P. Green DC330.00, One Hospital Drive, Columbia, Mo. 65212; 1-877-882-6826).

CHAPTER 10

Specific Exercises

•

In this chapter we will present examples of the three types of exercise prescribed for persons with rheumatoid arthritis (RA).

We have illustrated only one way to perform a given exercise, but there are many possibilities for each one. For example, a majority of the exercises illustrated in a standing position can be performed while sitting or lying down. Many people even perform their range-of-motion exercises before they get out of bed in the morning. This may be important for you if your hips, knees, ankles, or feet are affected by arthritis. You may want to get a sense of how the exercise feels standing and then try to duplicate the same motions while sitting or lying down. It is also possible to perform all your range-of-motion exercises in water. This is a wonderful way to get the benefits of buoyancy, as water sometimes makes it possible to perform exercises that otherwise cannot be done because of pain.

Strengthening exercises can also be performed in a variety of ways. You can do most of them sitting or lying. We use an exercise band for strengthening, but there are many ways to obtain the same type of resistance without using one. We have mentioned several alternatives in the text.

These exercises need not be performed in any particular order, although an exercise regimen should always begin with range-of-motion or stretching exercises. For instance, you may want to do several range-of-motion exercises first and then do some strengthening exercises. Or, you may want to perform exercises joint by joint (always beginning with some range-of-motion or stretching exercises). Some people like to do all of the floor exercises first and then move on to the sitting ones before performing the standing exercises last. Other people combine exercises. It's a good idea to try different approaches so you can discover a series of exercises that is comfortable for you.

If you do not have arthritis in some of the joints mentioned, you can bypass those exercises.

There are many range-of-motion, strengthening, and endurance exercises to choose from. Before you do any, please read Chapter 9, which provides guidelines about which types of exercises are best suited for your degree of inflammation. And keep the following guidelines and precautions in mind.

1. Review your exercise program with your physician or a **physical therapist** who is knowledgeable about RA. This is always important, but it is *crucial* if arthritis affects your neck or if your arthritis is severe. Take this book with you when you visit your doctor or therapist, and ask your doctor or therapist to check off the exercises that are best suited for your level of arthritis. You will also want the therapist or doctor to help you decide the number of repetitions of each exercise to perform. We have placed a box (□) near each exercise heading to help you keep a record of the recommended ones, and blank lines (_____) so you can write down the number of repetitions.
2. Make exercise a part of your daily routine.
3. Try to make exercise fun. Performing exercises with a friend or group makes exercise sessions more enjoyable. Your favorite music playing in the background can set the tone for exercising.
4. Exercise whenever you need to get "the kinks" out. Doing a brief series of range-of-motion and stretching exercises is excellent in the morning, for example, or when you have been sitting for long periods. These exercises decrease stiffness in the joints.
5. A formal exercise program with range-of-motion (and strengthening and endurance exercises if appropriate) should be done when your energy level is at its peak.
6. Balance your exercise program with adequate rest and sleep.
7. Always follow the rules of joint protection (see Chapter 8).
8. Be comfortable when you exercise:
   · Wear loose clothing.
   · Shower before exercising if you need to decrease pain and stiffness and increase flexibility.
   · Take arthritis medications in advance, timed to "kick in" during the exercise period.
9. Take deep, regular breaths while exercising. Remember, muscles use more oxygen than usual during exercise.
10. Use smooth, flowing movement. Avoid jerking or bouncing motions.
11. To limit inflammation, apply ice packs to warm joints for twenty minutes following an exercise session.
12. *Never* try to perform an exercise that causes pain. If it hurts, do not do it. (Forget the "no pain, no gain" philosophy.)
13. *Never* exercise to the point of extreme muscle fatigue or weakness.
14. If you have pain in your *joints* for more than two hours after exercising or notice increased *joint* pain or swelling the next day, you

are overdoing it. Cut back! On the other hand, some *muscle* soreness is expected when you first begin any exercise program.

15. If you have had joint replacements, always review exercises with your doctors, including your **orthopedic surgeon,** before proceeding.
16. Be adaptable to changes in your condition and modify accordingly.
17. Keep a log of exercises you have completed.

Range-of-Motion and Strengthening Exercises

If you have arthritis in your neck, consult your physician before attempting any of the following exercises. STOP IMMEDIATELY if you experience increased neck pain, dizziness, lightheadedness, numbness, or weakness in the arms or legs.

Neck Range-of-Motion Exercises

☐ **Exercise 1. Neck Stretch and Flexion**

Starting position: Sitting upright in a chair with your shoulders straight (A).

Step 1: While you are facing straight ahead pull your chin back; hold your chin in place for two to three seconds (B); relax.

Step 2: With your chin tucked in, slowly tilt your head forward toward your chest until you feel the muscles tighten in the back of your neck (C). Do not let your head drop downward. Hold your neck flexed for two to three seconds.

Repeat this exercise ____ times, ____ times per day.

☐ **Exercise 2. Neck Lateral Flexion**

Starting position: Sitting or standing, facing forward.

Step 1: Remain facing forward as you tilt your head sideways toward your right shoulder. Do not lift your right shoulder. Hold for two to three seconds.

Step 2: Return to the starting position.

Step 3: Repeat, tilting to the left side.

Repeat this exercise ____ times, ____ times per day.

☐ **Exercise 3. Neck Rotation**

Starting position: Sitting or standing, facing forward.

Step 1: Turn your head as though you were looking over your left shoulder. Hold for two to three seconds. Hold your shoulders straight, and do not let them turn with your head.

Step 2: Return to the center position.

Step 3: Repeat the exercise in the opposite direction.

Repeat this exercise ____ times, ____ times per day.

Neck Muscle-Strengthening Exercises

☐ **Exercise 4. Neck Extensor Strengthening**

Starting position: Standing or sitting with your back against a wall.

Step 1: Place the back of your head against the wall.

Step 2: Push your head back against the wall.

Step 3: Hold for six seconds, and then relax.

Repeat this exercise ____ times, ____ times per day.

☐ **Exercise 5. Neck Flexor Strengthening**

Starting position: Standing or sitting.

Step 1: Place the flat of your palm against your forehead.

Step 2: Push your head forward, opposing the resistance of your palm. Do not let your palm or your head move the other.

Step 3: Hold for six seconds, and then relax.

Alternatives: If arthritis in your elbow, hand, or wrist presents a problem, use a beach ball or pillow to provide resistance against your forehead.

Repeat this exercise _____ times, _____ times per day.

☐ **Exercise 6. Neck Lateral Flexor Strengthening**

Starting position: Standing or sitting.

Step 1: Place the flat of your right palm against the right side of your head.

Step 2: Push your head sideways against your right hand, resisting any movement of either.

Step 3: Hold for six seconds, and then relax.

Step 4: Repeat on left side.

Alternatives: If arthritis in your elbow, hand, or wrist presents a problem, use your upper arm, a beach ball, or a pillow as resistance against the tilting motion of your neck.

Repeat this exercise _____ times, _____ times per day.

Shoulder Range-of-Motion Exercises

☐ **Exercise 7. Shoulder Rotation**

Starting position: Standing, leaning forward with one hand placed against a table for support.

Step 1: Swing your opposite arm in small circles, rotating from the shoulder.

Step 2: Slowly increase the size of circles.

Step 3: Reverse arms.

Repeat this exercise ____ times, ____ times per day.

☐ Exercise 8. Shoulder Abduction and Adduction

Starting position: Standing or sitting with your arms at your sides.

Step 1: With your palms facing upward, swing your arms up along the side of your body until your hands touch above your head.

Step 2: Swing your arms back down to your sides.

Repeat this exercise ____ times, ____ times per day.

☐ Exercise 9. Shoulder Flexion and Extension

Starting position: Standing or sitting with your arms at your sides.

Step 1: Swing your left arm forward and your right arm backward simultaneously.

Step 2: Return your arms to your sides.

Step 3: Swing your right arm forward and your left arm backward.

Repeat this exercise ____ times, ____ times per day.

☐ Exercise 10. Shoulder External Rotation and Scapular Adduction; Internal Rotation

Starting position: Standing or sitting with your arms out at your sides.

Step 1: With your elbows bent and your fingers pointing upward and palms turned forward, pull your shoulders back, trying to squeeze your shoulder blades together (A); hold for two to three seconds.

Step 2: Keeping your elbows bent, bring your forearms to the front of your body, and try to make your hands and elbows meet (B).

Repeat this exercise ____ times, ____ times per day.

☐ **Exercise 11. Wall Walk**

Starting position: Standing, facing a wall, an arm's length away.

Step 1: Slowly walk the fingers of one hand up the wall.

Step 2: Step closer to the wall as you walk the fingers farther up it; hold for three seconds at the maximal height, pushing your armpit toward the wall.

Step 3: Observe how close your feet are to the wall so that you can monitor your progress.

Repeat this exercise _____ times, _____ times per day.

Elbow Range-of-Motion Exercises

☐ **Exercise 12. Elbow Extension and Flexion**

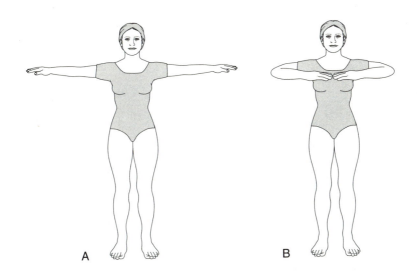

A   B

Starting position: Standing with your arms straight out from your sides, palms facing down.

Step 1: Hold your arms out, keeping your elbows straight (A).

Step 2: Bend your arms at the elbows, bringing your hands together in front of your body (B).

Repeat this exercise _____ times, _____ times per day.

☐ **Exercise 13. Elbow Pronation and Supination**

Starting position: Standing or sitting with your elbows bent and your fingers relaxed but pointing upward.

Step 1: Hold your arms up, turning your palms to face forward (A).

Step 2: Turn your hands so that the palms face backward (B).

A   B

Alternatives: If this causes you shoulder discomfort, perform the exercise while you are sitting with elbows supported on a table.

Repeat this exercise _____ times, _____ times per day.

Shoulder and Elbow Muscle-Strengthening Exercises

☐ **Exercise 14. Shoulder Abductor Strengthening**

Starting position: Standing, with an exercise band encircling your forearms.

Step 1: Separate your arms slowly, until you feel a firm pressure with the band tightening around your forearms.

Step 2: With your elbows straight, continue to push both arms out sideways against the band, resisting movement in the direction of either arm.

Step 3: Hold the muscle contraction for six seconds, then relax.

Alternatives: This exercise can be initiated with the band encircling your arms above the elbows. As your strength increases, the band can be lowered down your arm.

Repeat this exercise _____ times, _____ times per day.

☐ Exercise 15. Shoulder Flexor and Extensor Strengthening

Starting position: Standing, with an exercise band encircling your forearms.

Step 1: Raise your left arm and lower your right arm until you feel a firm pressure from the tightening band.

Step 2: Keeping your elbows straight, pull your left arm upward and push your right arm downward, resisting the pressure of the band.

Step 3: Hold the muscle contraction for six seconds, then relax.

Step 4: Repeat steps 1 through 3, reversing the arm motion.

Repeat this exercise _____ times, _____ times per day.

☐ Exercise 16. Shoulder External Rotator Strengthening

Starting position: Standing, with an exercise band encircling your forearms.

Step 1: Keeping your elbows pressed to your side, move your hands away from each other until you feel the band tighten around your forearms.

Step 2: Push outward with both forearms (keeping your elbows pressed tightly against your sides), resisting the pressure of the band.

Step 3: Hold the contraction for six seconds, then relax.

Repeat this exercise _____ times, _____ times per day.

☐ Exercise 17. Shoulder Internal Rotator Strengthening

Starting position: Stand with your elbows bent at your sides, with your forearms against your chest.

Step 1: Press your forearms against your chest while
holding your elbows in position.

Step 2: Hold the muscle contraction for six seconds,
then relax.

Repeat this exercise ____ times, ____ times per day.

☐ **Exercise 18. Elbow Flexor and Extensor
Strengthening**

Starting position: Standing, with an exercise band
encircling your forearms. (If you are using an elastic
trouser belt, you may have to double it up.)

Step 1: With your elbows bent, move your left
forearm upward and your right arm downward
until you feel the band tighten firmly around
your forearms.

Step 2: Pull your left forearm upward and push
your right downward, resisting the pressure of
the band.

Step 3: Hold the muscle contraction for six
seconds, then relax.

Step 4: Repeat steps 1 through 3, reversing the
motion of each arm.

Repeat this exercise ____ times, ____ times per
day.

Wrist and Finger Range-of-Motion Exercises

☐ **Exercise 19. Wrist
Extension and Flexion**

Step 1: Bend your wrist up as
though you were waving to
someone (A).

Step 2: Bend your wrist
downward as far as you
comfortably can (B).

Repeat this exercise ____ times,
____ times per day.

A

B

☐ Exercise 20. Wrist Medial and Lateral Flexion

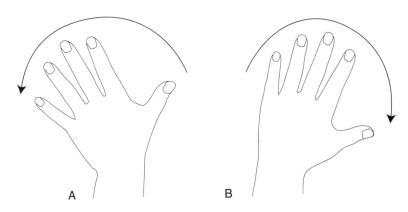

A   B

Step 1: With elbows bent and palms facing inward or forward, bend both wrists sideways in the direction of your little finger (A).

Step 2: Bend both wrists sideways in the direction of your thumb (B).

Repeat this exercise ____ times, ____ times per day.

☐ Exercise 21. Finger Walk

Step 1: Touch your thumb to your index finger (A).

A

Step 2: Touch your thumb to your middle finger (B).

Step 3: Touch your thumb to your ring finger (C).

B

Step 4: Touch your thumb to your little finger (D).

Repeat this exercise ____ times, ____ times per day.

C

D

☐ Exercise 22. Finger Flexion and Extension

Starting position: Begin by warming up with a finger walk (Exercise 21).

Step 1: Slowly curl your fingers, beginning at the tips and progressing down the knuckles until you form a loose fist (A).

Step 2: Uncurl your fingers, completely straightening and spreading them (B).

Repeat this exercise ____ times, ____ times per day.

A

B

Hip Range-of-Motion Exercises

☐ **Exercise 23. Hip Flexion and Extension**

Starting position: Standing, with right hand placed on a counter or table for balance.

Step 1: Swing your left leg forward, keeping your knee as straight as possible.

Step 2: Swing your left leg backward.

Step 3: Slowly increase the length of the swing until slight discomfort occurs. Do not let your leg's acceleration swing it beyond the painful limit.

Step 4: Turn around, place left hand on surface, and repeat with your right leg.

Repeat this exercise ____ times, ____ times per day.

☐ **Exercise 24. Hip Abduction**

Starting position: Standing, with your right hand resting on a counter for balance.

Step 1: Slowly swing your left leg outward and return it to the starting position.

Step 2: Turn around, place left hand on counter, and repeat with your right leg.

Repeat this exercise ____ times, ____ times per day.

☐ **Exercise 25. Hip Rotation**

Starting position: Standing, with right hand placed against a support.

Step 1: Holding your knee straight, make small circles with your left leg, rotating from the hip.

Step 2: Gradually increase the size of the circles.

Step 3: Turn around, support with left hand, and repeat steps 1 and 2 with your right leg.

Repeat this exercise ____ times, ____ times per day.

☐ **Exercise 26. Hip External and Internal Rotation**

A   B

Starting position: Standing, with right hand resting on a support.

Step 1: With your left knee bent and lifted, swing your left leg outward (A).

Step 2: Swing your left leg inward, bringing it in front of your right leg (B).

Step 3: Turn around, support with left hand, and repeat with your right leg.

Alternatives: Similar movements can be performed while you are sitting or lying on your back.

Repeat this exercise ____ times, ____ times per day.

☐ **Exercise 27. Hip Flexion with Hip and Knee Muscle Strengthening**

This exercise is more advanced than other range-of-motion exercises. Be sure to start slowly at first, and cut back on repetitions or discontinue this exercise if knee or hip discomfort occurs.

Starting position: Lying flat on your back.

Step 1: With left leg bent, lift your right leg slowly upward, keeping the knee straight. Don't lift higher than left knee.

Step 2: Lower your leg, slowly if you want maximum strengthening.

Step 3: Straighten left leg, bend right leg, and repeat, lifting left leg.

Step 4: Increase the height of leg elevation gradually.

Repeat this exercise _____ times, _____ times per day.

Knee Range-of-Motion Exercises

☐ **Exercise 28. Knee Flexion**

Starting position: Standing, resting your hands on a support.

Step 1: Bending your left knee, raise your left heel upward behind you.

Step 2: Lower your left heel slowly.

Step 3: Repeat with your right leg.

Alternatives: You can perform knee flexion while sitting down or lying on your stomach.

Repeat this exercise _____ times, _____ times per day.

□ **Exercise 29. Knee Extension**

Starting position: Sitting in a chair, with your feet flat on the floor.

Step 1: Slowly elevate your left lower leg to a horizontal position.

Step 2: Slowly lower your left leg.

Step 3: Repeat with your right leg.

Repeat this exercise ____ times, ____ times per day.

Hip and Knee Muscle-Strengthening Exercises

□ **Exercise 30. Hip and Knee Muscle Strengthening**

Starting position: Lying on your back, with an exercise band encircling your lower legs.

Step 1: Lift your right leg without bending your knee until you feel the band tighten around your lower legs. If you have lifted your leg more than six inches, the band is too large in diameter.

Step 2: Elevate your right leg while resisting motion by keeping your left leg on the floor or bed.

Step 3: Hold the muscle contraction for six seconds.

Step 4: Repeat steps 1 through 3 with opposite legs.

Repeat this exercise ____ times, ____ times per day.

□ **Exercise 31. Hip Abductor Strengthening**

Starting position: Lying on your back, with an exercise band encircling lower legs.

Step 1: Slowly spread your legs apart until you feel a firm pressure from the bands around your legs.

Step 2: Push each leg outward, resisting pull of the opposite leg.

Step 3: Hold the muscle contraction for six seconds.

Repeat this exercise ____ times, ____ times per day.

☐ **Exercise 32. Knee Extensor and Flexor Strengthening**

Starting position: Sitting in a chair with your back held straight and an exercise band encircling your lower legs (legs far enough apart to hold the band in place but not farther than hip width). Your feet are on the floor.

Step 1: Slowly raise your left lower leg, pushing upward against the resistance of the band.

Step 2: Hold the muscle contraction for six seconds.

Step 3: Repeat steps 1 and 2 with other leg.

Repeat this exercise ____ times, ____ times per day.

Ankle Range-of-Motion Exercises

☐ **Exercise 33. Ankle Flexion and Extension**

Starting position: Sitting, with your feet dangling.

Step 1: Bend your ankles, pulling your toes toward you; hold for two to three seconds; relax.

Step 2: Bend your ankles, pointing your toes away from you; hold for two to three seconds.

Alternatives: This exercise may also be performed while lying down.

Repeat this exercise _____ times, _____ times per day.

☐ **Exercise 34. Ankle Rotation**

Starting position: Sitting, with your feet dangling.

Step 1: Draw an imaginary circle with each ankle.

Step 2: Gradually increase the size of the circle.

Alternatives: This exercise may also be performed while lying down.

Repeat this exercise _____ times, _____ times per day.

Endurance, or Aerobic, Exercises

It is essential that you consult your doctor before beginning any aerobic exercise program.

When your arthritis is controlled and your joint flexibility is at its optimum and your muscles are strengthened, you are ready to begin improving your stamina. Aerobic exercise will enhance your fitness by improving your heart and lung function as well as circulation.

To gain aerobic benefits from your exercise, you must (1) raise your heart rate (beats per minute) to a conditioning level known as the *target heart rate;* (2) maintain your target heart rate for fifteen to thirty minutes in each aerobic session; (3) perform your aerobic program at least three times each week.

These three principles are your *goal,* not where you will be at the start. However, benefits can be gained from an aerobic program from the very beginning. If aerobic exercise is new to you, begin your program slowly. In time you will be fit enough to satisfy all three of the principles.

Trying to perform too much aerobic exercise too soon is counterproductive. You may experience extreme fatigue, shortness of breath, dizziness, and increased joint pain. *Don't overdo it.*

What Is Your Target Heart Rate?

Your *target heart rate* is the heart rate required for exercise to produce cardiovascular benefits. It is based primarily on your age. Determining your target heart rate requires some calculation, with your *maximal heart rate* being the first computation. (This is the highest heart rate that is safe for individuals of your age.) Your *target* heart rate is calculated to be 70 percent of your *maximal* rate. **Warning: Do *not* exercise at your *maximal* heart rate.**

To calculate your *maximal* heart rate, use the following formula: 220 minus your age equals your maximal heart rate. To calculate your *target* heart rate, multiply the maximal heart rate by 0.70 (which represents 70 percent). By way of example, suppose you are 60 years old. You would calculate your target heart rate in the following way:

$$220 - 60 = 160 \text{ (maximal heart rate)}$$
$$160 \times 0.70 = 112 \text{ (target heart rate)}$$

Hence, the target heart rate for someone who is 60 years of age would be 112.

If you are taking medications called beta blockers or calcium channel blockers, these formulas will not work for you. These medications are generally prescribed for high blood pressure or heart problems and can lower the heart rate. If you are on one of these medications, discuss your target heart rate with your doctor.

Taking Your Pulse

To find out what your *actual heart rate* is, you must learn to take your pulse. Turn your hand over so that you are looking at your left palm (Figure 16). Use the tips of your right index, middle, and ring fingers to feel for the pulse. Place your fingertips at the base of your thumb on the bone at the edge of your wrist. Then, slowly slide your fingertips toward the middle of the wrist, feeling for a pulsation. (If you feel tendons, you have gone too far.) You'll need practice to learn how much pressure to exert. Too much pressure will stop the pulse. Not enough pressure will prevent you from feeling it. Practice by using different degrees of firmness. You may also take your pulse in your right arm using the fingers of your left hand.

Once you find the pulse, you will need to count the pulsations to get your heart rate. Look at a watch or clock that measures seconds. Count the number of pulsations occurring in a fifteen-second period. Then, multiply that number by four. This will give you your actual heart rate in beats per minute.

For your convenience, the following chart lists some target heart rates for various ages as well as the number of pulsations you should count at your wrist in a fifteen-second period if you have reached your target heart rate. If you like, select the row that is closest to your age and use that number as your target rate.

Figure 16. Taking a pulse

Age (years)	Target Heart Rate (beats per minute)	Wrist Pulse (beats in 15 seconds)
20	140	35
25	137	34
30	133	33
35	130	32
40	126	31
45	122	30
50	119	30
55	116	29
60	112	28
65	108	27
70	105	26
75	101	25

Beginning Your Aerobic Exercise Program

Selecting a form of aerobic exercise depends on several factors: convenience, time constraints, the joints that are affected with arthritis, and most importantly, the form of exercise you enjoy. Possibilities include brisk walking, swimming, stationary bicycling, low-impact aerobics or dancing, cross-country skiing, and rowing. After you have chosen a program and your doctor has approved it, we recommend that you follow these guidelines when beginning:

· Always warm up for at least five to ten minutes with range-of-motion and stretching exercises.
· Start slowly in the beginning. Try five minutes of aerobic exercise the first day, checking your pulse before and after. If your pulse exceeds the target rate, slow down.
· Increase the time spent doing aerobic exercise by small increments each session. Alternating spurts of five minute high-intensity exercise with low-intensity rest periods is a good way to increase the duration of aerobic exercise. As you get in better condition, shorten and eliminate the rest periods until you can do fifteen to thirty minutes of uninterrupted aerobic exercise. In the beginning you should check your pulse at least every five minutes.
· *Stop immediately if you develop chest pain, palpitations, dizziness, shortness of breath, extreme fatigue, weakness, or increased joint pain.*
· If you have pain for more than two hours after exercise or experience increased joint pain or swelling the following day, modify the program.
· Always follow aerobic exercise with at least five minutes of cool-down exercise, allowing your heart rate and breathing to return to normal.

Guidelines for Specific Aerobic Exercise

Swimming or aquatic therapy. Your local chapter of the Arthritis Foundation may be able to recommend an arthritis aquatic program close to you. Roxanne McNeal, of the Aquatic Therapy Services in Abingdon, Maryland, has the following advice:

· Pool temperatures of 92° to 98°F are suitable for range-of-motion and stretching exercises but *not* for active aerobics. (Contact the management at the pool where you plan to exercise and ask what the temperature range of their pool is.)
· Pool temperatures of 82° to 86°F are best for aerobic exercise. Doing aerobics in higher pool temperatures can cause the body temperature to increase and blood vessels to dilate, resulting in lightheadedness.
· Avoid pool therapy if you have an open wound, a fever, severe low or high blood pressure, or a history of uncontrolled seizures.
· Breathe regularly from the diaphragm throughout the exercise.

Bicycling

· Adjust your seat high enough to have your legs almost fully straighten out when pedaling.
· Do not ride a bike with the handlebars too far away from the seat. This increases stress on the lower back, shoulders, elbows, and wrists.

· If you can adjust the pedal tension, keep it at the lowest level, to limit stress on your knees.
· Indoor cycles with arm motion attachments can decrease stress on the knees and still provide a good aerobic workout.
· Try out various models of stationary bikes (at a gym) or outdoor bicycles (at a bicycle shop) before purchasing one.
· Cooling down with light pedaling can be substituted for a range-of-motion cool-down.

Walking

· If you have severe arthritis of the knees or hips, walking may not be for you. Consider swimming or biking.
· Soak your feet in warm water, doing some gentle foot range-of-motion exercises before walking, to loosen up joints.
· Perform hip and knee range-of-motion exercises to stretch muscles in preparation for walking.
· Walk on a flat, level, relatively firm surface.
· Wear supportive walking shoes or athletic sneakers with good shock absorption capability.
· Swing your arms for balance while walking.
· In inclement weather, walk in a shopping mall or indoor track. Many malls have walking clubs you can join.
· If your feet are warm after walking, soak them in cool water for ten minutes.

For More Information

The Arthritis Foundation sponsors the following exercise courses and programs: Walk With Ease, PACE (People with Arthritis Can Exercise), and Arthritis Foundation Aquatic Program. Books and videotapes (of these programs) are available for home use. Contact your local Arthritis Foundation for more information.

A well-written book (by two Australians), containing complete exercise routines, is *Exercise Beats Arthritis: An Easy-to-Follow Program of Exercises,* by Valerie Sayce and Ian Frasier (Boulder, Colo.: Bull Publishing, 1998), which can be ordered at 1-800-676-2855 and *www.bullpub.com.*

Excellent resources by nationally recognized fitness leader Betty Perkins-Carpenter include a comprehensive low-impact program, *How to Prevent Falls: A Comprehensive Guide to Better Balance* (Senior Fitness Productions, 1989, 1991, 1993, 1999) and a stretching pamphlet, "Stretching in Bed" (Senior Fitness Productions, 2001), both of which can be ordered at 1-800-306-3137 and *www.senior-fitness.com.*

PART IV

Medications

•

CHAPTER 11

Medications Past, Present, Future

•

Taking medications can be inconvenient, and few medications are free of potential side effects. In the treatment of rheumatoid arthritis (RA), however, the benefits of medication almost always outweigh their inconvenience and risk. Medications decrease inflammation and prevent the permanent damage that can occur when RA is not brought under control. They can also help control pain. In short, medications are an *essential* ingredient in the treatment of RA.

In this chapter we examine how approaches to treatment, especially pharmaceutical treatment, have changed in response to new information emerging from medical research and experience. Then, in Chapters 12, 13, 14, and 15, we describe the three major groups of medications used today for treating RA and discuss how to take them, when to take them, when *not* to take them, and what their benefits and potential side effects are. Chapter 16 addresses the prevention and treatment of osteoporosis.

The Past: The Conservative Approach

Traditionally, medical therapy for RA was outlined according to a pyramid approach (Figure 17). Treatment options started at the base of the pyramid. Doctors would begin conservatively, by prescribing what was thought to be the safest medication. From the 1940s through the 1960s this first-line therapy took the form of large doses of aspirin. In the 1970s and 1980s many new nonsteroidal anti-inflammatory drugs (**NSAIDs**) became available. Because they are convenient and often well tolerated (patients notice few side effects), NSAIDs have gradually replaced aspirin as the first line of therapy.

Also located on the base of the pyramid were other conservative forms of treatment such as rest, physical therapy, and diet. Because *early* RA was thought to be a purely inflammatory and reversible condition, doctors believed that anti-inflammatory therapy *alone* was justified. Before doctors

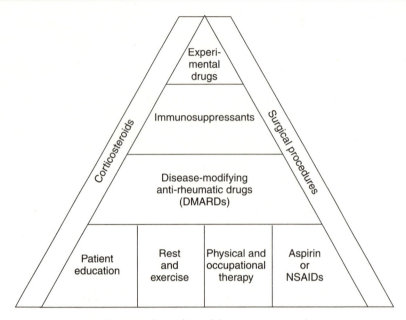

Figure 17. The traditional therapeutic pyramid

moved up to the next tier of treatment and prescribed second-line therapy, actual *damage* would need to be apparent by physical examination or x-ray. This was consistent with the theory of the time, which held that the early phase, the *inflammatory phase*, of RA was only *infrequently* followed by a more damaging *proliferative phase*. In this later phase, the **synovium** would become thicker and more destructive. Doctors often waited one to three years for evidence of this damaging phase before prescribing disease-modifying drugs (drugs that attempt to induce a remission by stopping the proliferative phase). These disease-modifying antirheumatic drugs (DMARDs), or *remittive* (causing **remission**) drugs, were thought to be unnecessary and too dangerous for early use.

The Present: More Aggressive Approaches to Therapy

The treatment of RA has changed dramatically in the past twenty years. Several important pieces of information have altered how we treat RA. First, it has been widely acknowledged that irreversible damage *can* take place during the first two years of RA, even before such damage is observed by standard x-rays. Second, we now know that, despite their effectiveness in decreasing inflammation, NSAIDs and COX-2 inhibitors do not change the course of RA, because they do not affect the proliferating, damaging synovium. Finally, DMARDs and **biologic response modifiers (BRMs)** (described below) appear to be most effective in *preventing* damage if they are used *early*. Hence, the old pyramid strategy, which postponed the most effective treatments until after damage was visible, has been abandoned by most rheumatologists for a more aggressive approach. This new strategy is commonly known among rheumatologists as "inverting the pyramid." Thus, most rheumatologists initiate disease-modifying medications (DMARDs) as soon as it is clear that a person has RA. The challenge today is to determine how early in the course of RA we should use our most powerful new biologic response modifiers.

The Future

In late 1998, we took a giant step into the future treatment of rheumatoid arthritis. After years of research, the first biogenetically engineered drug, Enbrel (etanercept) was made available to people with RA (more about this drug in Chapter 14). This drug is the first of a new class of drugs called the biologic response modifiers (BRMs). These medications are designed to target very specific parts of the immune system. Since 1998, other "biologics," Remicade, Kineret, and Humira, have been introduced, and more are on the way. The future will clearly bring efforts to identify the pivotal component of the immune system that has gone awry in RA and to correct it. This may involve the use of a single biologic drug or the use of a combination of more than one agent.

Current biologic therapies are directed against two inflammatory **cytokines, tumor necrosis factor (TNF)** and **interleukin-1 (IL-1)** (see Chapter 14). The future promises new biologic medications that will focus on blocking these two cytokines. Drug companies are developing biologics that are less expensive to manufacture and need to be taken less frequently. They are also looking at compounds that are even more selectively focused on blocking only the inflammatory aspects of these cytokines, leaving the beneficial aspects unaltered. Biologic treatments that can be delivered orally rather than by injection are in clinical trials. Suffice it to say that there are several companies looking at novel and improved ways of blocking these two critical inflammatory cytokines.

Scientists have identified several other inflammatory cytokines as targets for treatment (IL-6, IL-12, IL-15, and IL-17). Potential treatments aimed at these substances will increase our arsenal for fighting inflammation. Another small protein, called RANKL, has been identified. It activates bone-destroying cells called osteoclasts which may be responsible for the bone erosions that occur in RA. Studies looking at a natural

RANKL blocker (called OPG) are under way. If these treatments are effective, we have more options to prevent the damaging effects of RA on the bones and joints. Pharmaceutical and biotechnology companies are looking at dozens of different targets in the cascade of events responsible for RA.

The success of the Human Genome Project has made it possible to trace genes that may be linked to RA, and the future undoubtedly will bring novel drugs that exploit this new information. Whether these drugs will take the form of gene therapy or vaccines we do not yet know.

As we will discuss in Chapter 17, on nutrition, medical researchers are becoming more interested in the effects of diet on RA. There is an expanding scientific rationale for dietary management as an adjunct to traditional therapies. As we learn more about nutrition effects, we may begin to make dietary recommendations that can work in tandem with pharmaceuticals, biologics, and other therapies. All of this new information about RA makes us more hopeful about the future than ever before.

Current Treatments: NSAIDs, DMARDs, BRMs, and Corticosteroids

The four major groups of medications prescribed for the treatment of RA are:

1. NSAIDs. Nonsteroidal anti-inflammatory drugs are used to reduce inflammation quickly. This category also includes the new COX-2 inhibitors. (See Chapter 12.)
2. DMARDs. Disease-modifying antirheumatic drugs are used in an attempt to induce a remission. This category contains traditional DMARDs and immunosuppressants. (See Chapter 13.)
3. BRMs. Biologic response modifiers, a subset of DMARDs, are biogenetically engineered and usually given by injection or IV infusion. (See Chapter 14.)
4. Corticosteroids. Steroid anti-inflammatory medications are used to reduce inflammation. (See Chapter 15.)

We believe strongly that being aware of potential side effects from medications will help you recognize the symptoms early and will help ensure that you obtain prompt treatment if a side effect occurs. We would like to add a cautionary note about focusing too intently on the potential side effects of medications, however. Such a focus can cause unnecessary worry and stress. A proper balance is to be found somewhere between being aware of the symptoms of side effects and watching vigilantly for the possible occurrence of every one of them. Keep in mind that severe and irreversible side effects rarely happen.

As stated above, new medications become available continually. For this reason some drugs that are in use by the time you read this book may not be included in the following chapters. In any case, please consult your doctor for more information about medications.

A final note: We recommend that you use only one pharmacy to fill all of your prescriptions if possible. This allows the pharmacist to monitor the medications you are taking (possibly prescribed by more than one physician) and caution you and your physicians about potentially harmful drug interactions.

For More Information

The Arthritis Foundation offers free brochures about most drugs used in the treatment of rheumatoid arthritis. To order brochures, call 1-800-283-7800.

CHAPTER 12

Aspirin, Nonsteroidal Anti-inflammatory Drugs (NSAIDs), and COX-2 Inhibitors

·

Nonsteroidal anti-inflammatory drugs (**NSAIDs**) are among the most commonly prescribed drugs worldwide. These medications are classified as *anti-inflammatory* because they reduce pain and swelling quickly. They are classified as *nonsteroidal* because they are not included in the corticosteroid (cortisone) family of medications (see Chapter 13), which are also anti-inflammatory agents.

Aspirin and NSAIDs (pronounced *en'-seds* or *en'-sayds*) are used to treat a wide variety of inflammatory and painful conditions. With few exceptions, these medications work by arresting the production of the inflammatory substances known as prostaglandins (discussed in Chapter 1). Aspirin and NSAIDs can reduce pain, swelling, and stiffness in the joints by limiting the production of these chemicals.

These medications usually produce results within one to three weeks of first use, and therefore they are termed *fast-acting* or *rapid-acting* anti-arthritic drugs. They are generally the first line of treatment for rheumatoid arthritis (RA). Despite their effectiveness in controlling *symptoms,* these drugs do not appear to alter the course of the disease itself. In other words, they do *not* induce a remission of RA. Given this fact, your doctor may prescribe one or more second-line drugs along with anti-inflammatory medication, in an effort to induce a remission. (These slower-acting, disease-modifying drugs are described in Chapter 13.)

Several types and brands of anti-inflammatory drugs are now available, and many more are currently being tested. Finding the medication that will benefit you the most may take some time and experimentation. One may give you little relief, whereas another may be extremely effective. One may produce unpleasant side effects (such as indigestion), whereas another does not. Sometimes only by trying several medications, one at a time, can you determine which anti-inflammatory medication will help you the most. The latest addition to the NSAID family is the COX-2 inhibitor subset of anti-inflammatory drugs. COX-2 inhibitors appear to cause fewer side effects, particularly stomach irritation and ulceration.

Anti-inflammatory medications vary widely in cost as well as in effectiveness. A difference in cost is found between two forms of the same drug: these two forms are the *generic,* or non–brand name drug, and the brand name drug. The generic version will be the less expensive. Generic medications contain the same active ingredients found in brand name drugs, but the inactive ingredients may differ. Although these drugs may be as effective as the brand name counterpart, the quality in the production of brand name drugs has traditionally been more closely controlled, and therefore brand name drugs tend to be more consistent in their effectiveness. There is no evidence that generic arthritis drugs have more side effects than brand name medications, however, and if the expense of medications is a critical factor for you, you might want to consult your physician or pharmacist regarding the advisability of selecting a generic version or a less expensive medication.

Aspirin

Aspirin (acetylsalicyclic acid) is an extraordinarily effective medication that is often underestimated by patients and physicians alike. It is actually the standard against which all other anti-inflammatory drugs are compared. We underrate its value because it is inexpensive, available without a prescription, and easily obtained. In addition to decreasing inflammation, aspirin also decreases pain and fever. Few medications can boast as amazing a profile and successful a track record as aspirin.

Different doses of aspirin work differently; low doses of aspirin (one baby aspirin a day) provide some protection for people with heart problems, whereas one or two aspirins taken every four to six hours can relieve a fever or headache. For treating RA, we are interested in the anti-inflammatory effects of aspirin, which occur only with very large doses.

It is not uncommon for doctors to prescribe ten to twenty regular-strength aspirin tablets per day to control inflammation. Such large doses, called *high-dose aspirin therapy,* must be accompanied by routine monitoring of blood salicylate levels. The salicylate level in your blood must be adequate to control inflammation without being so high that it causes side effects such as ringing in the ears, or tinnitus. *Do not take large doses of aspirin unless you are under the supervision of a physician.*

Aspirin is available in several forms that span a wide price range. Every formulation contains the same active ingredient: aspirin. One aspirin product is no more effective than another as long as the dose and absorption are adequate, but differences in the formulations of aspirin products do affect the convenience of aspirin use and may have some bearing on the side effects produced as well.

Plain Aspirin

Over-the-counter brand name examples: Empirin, Norwich

This is the most economical form. Although aspirin is aspirin as far as effectiveness is concerned, aspirin that dissolves easily is less likely to settle near the stomach lining and irritate it. Hence, the very hard, compact tablet may not be as safe as a more powdery variety. Aspirin that smells like vinegar is old and should not be used.

Buffered Aspirin

Over-the-counter brand name examples: Arthritis Pain Formula,
    Ascriptin, Bufferin

Buffered aspirin contains an ingredient that partially neutralizes stomach acids. This form of aspirin may cause less stomach upset or indigestion than other forms, but it does not decrease the risk of developing **gastritis** (stomach irritation) or ulcer from aspirin use.

Film-Coated Aspirin

Over-the-counter brand name examples: Anacin, Bayer

A film or coating on the tablet makes it easier to swallow. This coating is not an enteric coating, nor does it protect the stomach in any way.

Enteric-Coated Aspirin

Over-the-counter brand name examples: Ecotrin, Entab-650
Prescription brand name example: Easprin

An enteric coating is applied which causes the tablets to pass through the stomach and into the small intestine before dissolving. There is evidence that this decreases the risk of stomach upset and direct irritation. The risk for gastritis and ulcers, although present, is slightly decreased with this formulation.

The slowly dissolving coating sometimes interferes with the body's ability to absorb this type of aspirin. There have also been reports that enteric aspirin is retained in the stomach of patients with sluggish digestive systems. If this form proves ineffective for you, your doctor may want to check the salicylate levels in your blood to determine whether you are adequately absorbing your medication.

Timed-Release Aspirin

Over-the-counter brand name example: Eight-hour Bayer Timed-
  Release
Prescription brand name examples: Encaprin, Zorprin

This controlled-release preparation gradually releases the aspirin. Because much of the aspirin is released after the tablet or capsule reaches the intestines (rather than in the stomach), this form may decrease stomach upset and indigestion. It does not eliminate the risks of gastritis or ulcer. Because it is taken fewer times during the day, it is more convenient, but it is significantly more expensive than regular aspirin.

Side Effects of Aspirin Therapy

The most common side effect of high-dose aspirin therapy is stomach distress (Table 1). Symptoms are usually minor and can be relieved by taking the aspirin with meals.

Another common side effect is blood passed in tiny amounts daily in the stool. This is usually not dangerous, but it can lead to **anemia.**

Table 1
Side Effects of Aspirin

Side Effects	Incidence	Side Effect Therapy
Nuisance		
Increased bleeding from cuts or tendency to bruise easily	Common	Unnecessary
Ear ringing or temporary changes in hearing	Common	Discontinue aspirin or reduce dosage
Nausea, indigestion, or heartburn	5–25%	Take aspirin with food, reduce dosage, or change medication
Serious		
Gastritis or stomach ulcers	Occasional	Discontinue aspirin and take stomach medication
Bleeding ulcers	Infrequent	Obtain prompt medical evaluation, discontinue aspirin, and take stomach medication
Abnormal liver tests	5%	Discontinue aspirin if markedly abnormal

Some people on high-dose aspirin therapy develop serious stomach problems, such as **gastritis** and stomach ulcer. Fortunately, bleeding ulcers are infrequent. Anyone developing one of these problems needs to stop taking aspirin and begin treatment with special stomach medications. The medication *misoprostol* (Cytotec) helps prevent these side effects. (See the end of this chapter for details about available stomach medications.)

Cautionary Notes

Before starting aspirin therapy, discuss the following with your physician:

· Any history of allergy to aspirin or other anti-inflammatory medications. Symptoms of allergy include rash, hives, and swollen lips or eyelids. Wheezing and difficulty with breathing are rare and serious allergic responses.
· A history of asthma, nasal polyps, stomach ulcer, bleeding problems, colitis, kidney or liver problems.
· Any medications that you are presently taking. Of particular importance are blood thinners, diabetes medication, blood pressure pills, seizure medication, and over-the-counter pain medications.

While taking aspirin:

· Contact your physician promptly if you notice dark or tar-colored bowel movements, persistent indigestion or nausea, stomach pain that is relieved by eating.
· Never take more than one anti-inflammatory drug at a time (aspirin counts as a drug). If your doctor prescribes a new NSAID, he or she will almost certainly take you off high-dose aspirin; if he or she fails to discuss this with you, you should ask about it. *Do not take over-the-counter anti-inflammatory medications such as ibuprofen, naproxen, or ketoprofen while you are taking high doses of aspirin.* If your physician approves, *acetaminophen* (Tylenol) may be taken while you are taking aspirin. Unless you are instructed otherwise, you should take aspirin at mealtime, to reduce indigestion and stomach irritation.
· Inform your dentist, surgeon, and anyone else performing health care procedures that you are on aspirin therapy.
· Avoid drinking alcohol and smoking, because these practices increase your risk of developing an ulcer.
· Your doctor may periodically request blood tests for blood cell counts, kidney and liver tests, and tests for electrolytes (sodium and potassium) levels, and may examine your stool for blood.

Pregnancy and breastfeeding. Aspirin should be avoided during pregnancy, particularly during the last trimester, unless specifically prescribed by your doctor. Aspirin therapy may affect the fetus or cause complications during labor and delivery.

Salicylates are excreted in breast milk, and therefore large doses of aspirin should be avoided while nursing.

Traditional NSAIDs

Like high doses of aspirin, NSAIDs can decrease pain, stiffness, and swelling in the joints. NSAIDs are generally more convenient to take than most forms of aspirin, and they generally cause less stomach upset. Since the first modern NSAID (indomethacin) was marketed in 1965, many more have become available; you probably are familiar with one or more of them (see Table 2).

Dosages of different NSAIDs are not comparable, that is, 1 milligram of one NSAID is not necessarily equal to 1 milligram of another NSAID. One 800-milligram pill of ibuprofen, for example, is nearly equivalent to a 75-milligram pill of the NSAID ketoprofen. *Dosages of NSAIDs should be determined and monitored by your physician.*

The following NSAIDs are commonly used in the treatment of RA. With the exception of ibuprofen, the NSAIDs described here are available only by prescription. (The scientific name of the drug comes first; the names in parentheses are proprietary brand names.)

Diclofenac (Voltaren, Voltaren XL, Cataflam)

Tablet size: 25, 50, 75 mg
Extended-release tablet size: 100 mg

Diclofenac is taken two to three times daily. Extended-release diclofenac is usually taken only once per day. The brand name version Voltaren has an enteric coating; because of this it tends to be well tolerated by the stomach. There is a question of slightly increased liver problems with diclofenac compared to other NSAIDs.

Diclofenac/misoprostol Combination (Arthrotec)

Tablet size: 50, 75 mg

Arthrotec is a combination pill that contains the NSAID diclofenac as well as a stomach-protecting medication. Arthrotec is usually taken twice per day. Because the tablet contains the stomach protector misoprostol, there is less chance of stomach problems.

Table 2
Nonsteroidal Anti-inflammatory Drugs (NSAIDs)

Drug	Brand Name	Generic Available?
Diclofenac	Voltaren	yes
	Voltaren XR	yes
	Cataflam	yes
Diclofenac/misoprostol	Arthrotec	no
Diflunisal	Dolobid	yes
Etodolac	Lodine	yes
	Lodine XL	yes
Fenoprofen	Nalfon	yes
Flurbiprofen	Ansaid	yes
Ibuprofen	Advil[a]	—
	Medipren[a]	—
	Midol[a]	—
	Motrin IB[a]	—
	Nuprin[a]	—
	Motrin	yes
Indomethacin	Indocin	yes
Ketoprofen	Orudis	yes
	Orudis KT[a]	—
	Actron[a]	—
	Oruvail	yes
Magnesium choline trisalicylate	Trilisate	yes
Meclofenamate	Meclomen	yes
Meloxicam	Mobic	no
Nabumetone	Relafen	yes
Naproxen	Naprosyn	yes
Naproxen sodium	Naprelan	yes
	Anaprox	yes
	Anaprox DS	yes
	Alleve[a]	—
Oxaprozin	Daypro	yes
Piroxicam	Feldene	yes
Salsalate	Disalcid	yes
Sulindac	Clinoril	yes
Tolmetin	Tolectin	yes

Note: Unless noted otherwise, these NSAIDs are available by prescription only.
[a] Available over the counter, without prescription.

Diflunisal (Dolobid)

Tablet size: 250, 500 mg

Diflunisal is taken twice daily. It differs from most other NSAIDs in being a close relative of the salicylate family, which includes aspirin. It is also one of the more effective NSAIDs for relieving pain.

Etodolac (Lodine)

Tablet size: 400, 500 mg
Extended-release tablet size: 400, 500 mg
Capsule size: 200, 300 mg

Etodolac is generally taken two to four times per day. Extended-release tablets are taken one to two times per day. Etodolac is generally well tolerated.

Fenoprofen (Nalfon)

Tablet size: 600 mg
Capsule size: 200, 300 mg

Fenoprofen is generally taken three or four times daily. There is a possibility of slightly increased risk of kidney problems with fenoprofen compared with other NSAIDs.

Flurbiprofen (Ansaid)

Tablet size: 50, 100 mg

Flurbiprofen is taken two or three times daily. It is an excellent pain reliever and causes comparatively fewer headaches than other NSAIDs.

Ibuprofen

Over-the-counter brand name examples: Advil, Medipren, Midol 200, Motrin IB, Nuprin
Tablet size: 200 mg

Prescription brand name examples: Motrin, Rufen
Tablet size: 300, 400, 600, 800 mg
Liquid form is available without prescription.

Ibuprofen is generally taken three or four times daily. It is available without a prescription. Ibuprofen is generally well tolerated and is a proven pain reliever. It has been approved by the Food and Drug Administration

(FDA) for use by children. For treatment of RA, the dosage of ibuprofen is greater than that recommended on the manufacturer's package. *Do not take large doses of ibuprofen without a physician's guidance.* In addition, to avoid increased toxicity, ibuprofen should not be taken with other NSAIDs.

Indomethacin (Indocin)

Capsule size: 25, 50 mg
Sustained-release capsule: 75 mg
Liquid and suppository forms are available.

Indomethacin is generally taken two or three times daily. The sustained-release capsule is taken once or twice per day. Indomethacin results in comparatively more headaches and stomach distress than other NSAIDs. It is generally considered one of the most potent NSAIDs in terms of anti-inflammatory effect.

Ketoprofen (Orudis, Oruvail)

Over-the-counter brand name examples: Actron, Orudis KT
Tablet size: 12.5 mg

Prescription brand name examples: Orudis, Oruvail (extended release)
Capsule size: 25, 50, 75 mg
Extended-release capsule size: 100, 150, 200 mg

Prescription ketoprofen is generally taken two or three times daily. Extended-release capsules are taken once per day. Ketoprofen appears to be an excellent pain reliever for many people. Take over-the-counter ketoprofen only with your doctor's knowledge. Do not take this medication with other NSAIDs even if it is an over-the-counter variety.

Magnesium Choline Trisalicylate (Trilisate)

Tablet size: 500, 750, 1000 mg
Liquid form is available.

This medication is taken two or three times daily. It differs from most other NSAIDs in being a close relative of the salicylate family, which includes aspirin. However, it is different from aspirin and other NSAIDs in some very important ways. It is one of the safer NSAIDs because it results in a very low incidence of stomach irritation and ulceration. It also has little or no effect on the kidneys and platelets. The trade-off for this wonderful safety profile is that it may not be as effective for pain relief as other NSAIDs. Like aspirin, it can also cause more ear ringing and reversible hearing loss than other NSAIDs. Salicylate levels in the blood are monitored to produce the most effective therapy possible.

Meclofenamate (Meclomen)

Capsule size: 50, 100 mg

Meclofenamate is generally taken three or four times daily. It is a very good pain reliever. Complaints of abdominal cramping and diarrhea, particularly when it is used in high doses, limit its continued use in some people.

Meloxicam (Mobic)

Tablet size: 7.5, 15 mg

Meloxicam became available in the United States in the year 2000. It had been used successfully in other countries for several years before then. Although not technically classified as a **COX-2 inhibitor,** it has many of the same characteristics. Compared to traditional NSAIDs, it appears to have a less irritating effect on the stomach.

Nabumetone (Relafen)

Tablet size: 500 mg

Nabumetone has a convenient once-a-day dosing. Released in 1992, this NSAID may cause fewer stomach problems than many other traditional NSAIDs.

Naproxen (Naprosyn)

Prescription brand name examples: Naprosyn, Naprosyn EC (enteric coated)
Tablet size: 250, 375, 500 mg
Enteric-coated tablet size: 375, 500 mg
Liquid form is available.

See description below.

Naproxen Sodium (Alleve, Anaprox, Naprelan)

Prescription brand name examples: Anaprox, Anaprox DS, Naprelan (extended release)
Tablet size: 250, 500 mg

Extended-release tablet size: 375, 500 mg

Over-the-counter brand name example: Alleve
Tablet size: 200 mg

Naproxen and naproxen sodium are convenient NSAIDs that are taken twice a day. The availability of an over-the-counter product has made this medication very popular. Both provide excellent pain relief. This medication should *not* be taken with other NSAIDs.

Oxaprozin (Daypro)

Tablet size: 600 mg

Oxaprozin is an NSAID that can be given once daily. The usual dosage is two tablets per day. Some individuals choose to divide the doses. This anti-inflammatory drug is very well tolerated by most individuals.

Phenylbutazone (Azolid, Butazolidin)

Tablet size: 100 mg
Capsule size: 100 mg

Phenylbutazone is rarely prescribed for RA today because of the unpredictable occurrence of bone marrow complications and the availability of safer NSAIDs.

Piroxicam (Feldene)

Capsule size: 10, 20 mg

Piroxicam's major virtue is its once daily dosage. Excellent compliance with this dosing schedule is usually possible. Because this medication stays in the body longer than other NSAIDs, it has to be monitored closely in certain individuals.

Salsalate (Disalcid)

Tablet size: 500, 750 mg
Capsule size: 500 mg

Salsalate is taken three or four times daily. It differs from other NSAIDs in that it is classified as being in the salicylate family of medications, which includes aspirin. However, it differs from aspirin and other NSAIDs in many respects. It is one of the safer NSAIDs because it results in a very low incidence of stomach irritation and ulceration. In addition, it has little or no effect on the kidneys and platelets. Unfortunately, this safe and effective anti-inflammatory drug may not relieve pain as well as other NSAIDs. Like aspirin and magnesium choline trisalicylate, it can cause comparatively more ear ringing and reversible hearing loss than other NSAIDs. Salicylate levels in the blood are monitored to produce the most effective therapy possible.

Sulindac (Clinoril)

Tablet size: 150, 200 mg

Sulindac has a simple twice daily dosage. It tends to be well tolerated. There also appears to be a *slight* decrease in the risk for kidney problems with this medication as compared with some other NSAIDs. However, there may exist a slight risk that gallbladder and pancreas problems may arise from its use.

Tolmetin (Tolectin)

Tablet size: 200, 600 mg
Capsule size: 400 mg

Tolmetin is usually taken three or four times daily. Its use sometimes results in a false reading of protein in the urine. This can be misleading, because one rare but real side effect of tolmetin and the other NSAIDs is protein in the urine. Tolectin has been approved by the FDA for use in children.

Side Effects of Traditional NSAIDs

The most common side effects of NSAIDs are stomach upset (see Table 3). These symptoms are generally relieved by taking the medication with a meal or by adjusting the dosage.

Patients who have been taking NSAIDs for a long time can develop serious stomach problems (**gastritis** or stomach ulcer). Bleeding ulcers are an infrequent side effect of NSAID therapy. If gastritis, stomach ulcer, or bleeding ulcer develop, however, you will need to discontinue taking the NSAID and take medication that treats your stomach problem. Again, misoprostol helps prevent this side effect. (Stomach medications are discussed at the end of this chapter.)

In 1999, the first of a new group of NSAIDs, called COX-2 inhibitors was introduced. This subset of NSAIDs should be considered for people who have experienced stomach problems or are considered at high risk for stomach problems or are considered at high risk for stomach irritation (see next section).

Table 3
Side Effects of NSAIDs

Side Effects	Incidence	Side Effect Therapy
Nuisance		
Heartburn, nausea, and stomach pain	Common	Take with food or try a different NSAID
Cramping or diarrhea	Common	Take with food or reduce dosage
Rash	3–9%	Discontinue NSAID
Fluid retention, weight gain, ankle swelling	Common	Decrease salt intake
Headache, drowsiness, dizziness, difficulty concentrating	Common	Discontinue NSAID or try a different NSAID
Increased bleeding from cuts or tendency to bruise easily	Common	Usually no treatment
Ear ringing or mild change in hearing	Common	Discontinue NSAID or reduce dosage
Serious		
Abnormal liver tests	3%	Discontinue NSAID or reduce dosage if markedly abnormal since hepatitis is a rare consequence of NSAID use
Gastritis or stomach ulcers	Occasional	Discontinue NSAID and take stomach medication
Bleeding ulcers	Infrequent	Obtain prompt medical evaluation, discontinue NSAID, and take stomach medication
Kidney problems	Infrequent	Discontinue NSAID
Blood problems	Rare	Discontinue NSAID

A less common side effect of NSAID therapy is kidney problems. Such problems are rare in healthy individuals, but some people have known risk factors for developing such problems. These include diabetes, uncontrolled high blood pressure, age greater than sixty, a history of kidney disease, significant liver disease, heart failure, and hardening of the arteries. Almost all kidney problems caused by NSAIDs resolve when the medication is discontinued.

Cautionary Notes

Before starting NSAID therapy, discuss the following with your physician:

· A history of allergy to aspirin or other anti-inflammatory medication. Symptoms of allergy include rash, hives, wheezing, and swollen lips or eyelids.
· Previous history of asthma, nasal polyps, stomach ulcer, bleeding problems, colitis, high blood pressure, or kidney or liver problems.
· Any medications you are taking, particularly medications for blood thinning, diabetes, gout, high blood pressure, pain, or seizures.

While taking NSAIDs:

· Contact your physician promptly if you notice dark or tar-colored bowel movements, persistent indigestion or nausea, stomach pain that is relieved by eating.
· Never take more than one NSAID at a time. If your doctor prescribes a new NSAID, he or she will almost certainly take you off the other; if the doctor fails to discuss this with you, you should ask about it. *Do not take over-the-counter anti-inflammatory medications, such as ibuprofen, ketoprofen, naproxen, or aspirin, while you are taking another NSAID.* If your physician approves, *acetaminophen* (Tylenol) may be taken while you are taking an NSAID.
· Unless you are instructed otherwise, you should take the NSAID at mealtime, to reduce indigestion and stomach irritation.
· Inform your dentist, surgeon, and anyone else performing health care procedures on you that you are taking an NSAID.
· Wait two to four weeks before judging the effectiveness of the NSAID.
· Avoid drinking alcohol and smoking, because these practices increase your risk of developing an ulcer.
· Your doctor may periodically request blood tests for blood cell counts, kidney and liver tests, and tests for electrolyte (sodium and potassium) levels, as well as examine your stool for blood.

Pregnancy and breastfeeding. Not all NSAIDs have been studied adequately as to their effects on pregnancy, but it is generally recommended that they be discontinued during pregnancy. Most NSAIDs are excreted to some degree in the breast milk, and hence their use is usually discouraged during nursing. The manufacturer's package insert can be reviewed by you and your physician for information about the use of a specific NSAID during pregnancy and nursing. Discuss all medications with your obstetrician and your pediatrician.

New NSAIDs: COX-2 Inhibitors

In December 1998 the FDA approved the first cyclo-oxygenase-2 inhibitor, the brand name Celebrex. In May 1999, a second COX-2 inhibitor, Vioxx, was released. Two others, Bextra and Arcoxia, are now available, and certainly more will follow. Milder on the stomach, these anti-inflammatory drugs are welcome additions to the pharmaceutical choices for people who cannot tolerate traditional NSAIDs.

Cyclo-oxygenase-2 or COX-2 is an enzyme in the body known to stimulate inflammation by producing **prostaglandins.** Some prostaglandins can cause pain and swelling. Both COX-2 inhibitors and traditional NSAIDs block ("inhibit") the COX-2 enzyme and limit the production of "inflammatory" prostaglandins, thereby decreasing symptoms of inflammation. Traditional NSAIDs also block COX-1, an enzyme known to protect the stomach lining by producing "protective" prostaglandins. Blocking the production of the good variety of prostaglandins can result in stomach irritation and possibly ulcers, as well as a higher risk of bleeding problems. Researchers at the University of Rochester discovered that they could create medications that could block the production of inflammatory prostaglandins (by blocking COX-2 enzyme) without interfering with the function of the protective prostaglandins (produced by COX-1 enzyme). The result was a safer class of NSAIDs, which were named COX-2 inhibitors. The availability of the COX-2 inhibitors has made it possible for many people who couldn't tolerate traditional NSAIDs to relieve their pain and swelling with less risk of stomach ulceration and bleeding. Although safer, this group of anti-inflammatory agents has not been proven to be more effective than traditional NSAIDs for relieving symptoms of arthritis. Also, these medications are not a replacement for the DMARDs, the disease-modifying antirheumatic drugs, which affect not just the symptoms but the disease itself.

Unlike traditional NSAIDs, COX-2 inhibitors can be cautiously pre-

Table 4
COX-2 Inhibitors

Drug	Brand Name	Generic Available
Celecoxib	Celebrex	no
Valdecoxib	Bextra	no
Rofecoxib	Vioxx	no
Enterocoxib	Arcoxia	no

scribed for people who are already taking blood thinners, such as Coumadin (warfarin). The doctor will want to monitor your blood tests closely to look for changes in a test called INR or Protime. The dose of your blood thinner may have to be adjusted while you are on both medications. Your physician may also choose to place you on low-dose aspirin while you are on a COX-2 inhibitor. This would depend on your individual risk for side effects, such as a history of bleeding ulcer. Many people will require low-dose aspirin if their personal history makes them at risk for heart attack or stroke.

Celecoxib (Celebrex)

Capsule size: 100, 200 mg

Celecoxib can be taken once or twice daily. Some find that taking the medication in the evening helps diminish morning stiffness. This anti-inflammatory agent is very effective and well tolerated. If you have an allergy to sulfa drugs, you may not be able to take this medication. Be sure to discuss *all* medication allergies with your physician before starting any new medication.

Enterocoxib (Arcoxia)

Arcoxia is anticipated to be available in 2003. It is expected to be similar to other COX-2 inhibitors in safety and effectiveness.

Rofecoxib (Vioxx)

Tablet size: 12.5, 25, 50 mg
Liquid form is available.

Rofecoxib is taken once a day. This medication is effective for pain relief and is well tolerated. The FDA recommends using the highest pill dose, 50 mg, for only very short periods (less than five days). Some physicians do cautiously prescribe this higher dose for longer periods, monitoring the patient closely for high blood pressure and fluid retention.

Valdecoxib (Bextra)

Tablet size: 10, 20 mg

Bextra is a once-a-day COX-2 inhibitor. Early studies suggest that it is effective and well tolerated by people with RA. If you have an allergy to sulfa drugs, you may not be able to take this medication.

Side Effects of COX-2 Inhibitors

The most common side effects of the COX-2 inhibitors are abdominal pain, nausea, indigestion, and diarrhea. There appears to be a slightly higher risk of high blood pressure and fluid retention, particularly at high dosages. Like traditional NSAIDs, there is a slight risk of irritating the kidneys or liver. Stomach ulceration and bleeding are less likely than with traditional NSAIDs. (See Table 5.)

Table 5
Side Effects of COX-2 Inhibitors

Side Effects	Incidence	Side Effect Therapy
Nuisance		
Heartburn, nausea, and stomach pain	Infrequent	Take with food or try different COX-2 inhibitor
Cramping or diarrhea	Occasional	Take with food
Rash	Infrequent	Discontinue medication
Fluid retention, weight gain, ankle swelling	Common	Reduce dose or decrease salt intake
Headache, drowsiness, dizziness, difficulty concentrating	Occasional	Discontinue medication
Ear ringing or mild change in hearing	Occasional	Discontinue medication or reduce dosage
Serious		
High blood pressure	Occasional	Discontinue medication or reduce dosage
Abnormal liver tests	Infrequent	Discontinue medication if severe
Gastritis or stomach ulcers	Infrequent	Discontinue medication and take stomach medication
Bleeding ulcers	Rare	Obtain prompt medical evaluation Discontinue medication and take stomach medication
Kidney problems	Infrequent	Discontinue medication
Blood clotting problems	Unknown at this time	Discuss latest research with your doctor

Cautionary Notes

Before starting a COX-2 inhibitor, discuss the following with your physician:

· History of uncontrolled high blood pressure, ankle swelling, or fluid retention
· History of sulfa allergy (particularly if considering celecoxib or valdecoxib)
· History of allergy to aspirin or other anti-inflammatory medications (symptoms include rash, hives, wheezing, swollen lips or eyelids)
· History of asthma, nasal polyps, stomach ulcer, colitis, or kidney or liver problems
· History of heart attack, stroke, or blood clots
· Any medications you are taking, particularly medications for blood thinning, gout, high blood pressure, pain, or seizures

While taking a COX-2 inhibitor:

· Contact your physician promptly if you notice dark or tar-colored bowel movements, persistent indigestion or nausea, or stomach pain that is relieved by eating.
· Never take more than one COX-2 inhibitor or NSAID at a time. If your doctor prescribes a COX-2 inhibitor, he or she will take you off other NSAIDs; if he or she fails to discuss this with you, you should ask. *Do not take COX-2 inhibitors with over-the-counter anti-inflammatory medications such as ibuprofen, ketoprofen, or naproxen. Read labels.* Ask your doctor about low-dose aspirin if you are on aspirin for other reasons. If your physician approves, acetaminophen (Tylenol) may be taken while you are on a COX-2 inhibitor.
· Inform your dentist, surgeon, and anyone else performing health care procedures that you are taking a COX-2 inhibitor.
· Avoid drinking alcohol and smoking, which increase your risk of developing an ulcer.
· Your doctor may periodically request blood tests for blood cell counts, kidney and liver tests, and tests for electrolyte (sodium and potassium) levels, as well as examine your stool for blood.

Pregnancy and breastfeeding. COX-2 inhibitors have not been studied adequately as to their effects on pregnancy. It is generally recommended that they be discontinued during pregnancy. Most COX-2 inhibitors are excreted to some degree in breast milk, and hence their use is usually discouraged during nursing. The manufacturer's package insert can be reviewed by you and your physician for information about the use of specific COX-2 inhibitors during pregnancy and nursing. Discuss all medications with your obstetrician and your pediatrician.

Table 6
Stomach Medications

Purpose of Drug	Drug Name	Brand Name
Prescription		
Prevents stomach ulcers; protects the stomach	Misoprostol	Cytotec
Decreases acid production	Cimetidine[a]	Tagamet
	Famotidine[a]	Pepcid
	Nizatidine[a]	Axid
	Ranitidine[a]	Zantac
	Prilosec[a]	Omeprazole
	Prevacid	Lansoprazole
	Protonix	Pantoprazole
	Nexium	Esomeprazole
	Aciphex	Rabeprazole
Coats the stomach	Sucralfate[a]	Carafate
Over-the-counter		
Neutralizes acids	Antacid	Mylanta
		Maalox
		Rolaids
		Tums
Decreases acid production	Cimetidine[b]	Tagamet[b]
	Famotidine[b]	Pepcid AC[b]
	Nizatidine[b]	Axid[b]

[a] Available in generic.
[b] Lower dosage than prescribed version of same drug.

Stomach Medications Frequently Used with NSAIDs

Because aspirin and NSAIDs can cause stomach problems such as gastritis and ulcers, it is sometimes necessary to take medications to treat these conditions. Stomach problems often can be relieved by changing from a traditional NSAID to a COX-2 inhibitor. If not, there are many other options for relieving stomach problems. Some of the stomach medications are listed in Table 6.

CHAPTER 13

Disease-Modifying
Antirheumatic Drugs (DMARDs)

•

The purpose of disease-modifying antirheumatic drugs (DMARDs) is to alter the course of rheumatoid arthritis (RA)—to control the arthritis process and prevent damage. DMARDs are also commonly referred to as *second-line* agents, because traditionally they were used only after NSAIDs or anti-inflammatory medications had failed. They are also occasionally known as *slow-acting antirheumatic drugs* (*SAARDs*), because it often takes several weeks to months before they begin to work.

All drugs that are classified as DMARDs have been *presumed* to be effective in slowing down the process of RA. In some cases they may even induce a complete remission of the condition (which explains why they are sometimes referred to as *remittive* drugs). Their ability to affect the course of RA distinguishes this group of drugs from NSAIDs, which effectively treat symptoms, such as pain and swelling, but do not change the course of the disease. Although traditional DMARDs do not provide fast pain relief, improved comfort is often a long-term benefit of using them to control the arthritis process.

Fourteen medications are considered by most rheumatologists to fit in the DMARD family. Seven of these medications—injectable gold, gold pills, hydroxychloroquine, penicillamine, sulfasalazine, leflunamide, and minocycline—are categorized strictly as DMARDs. We do not fully understand how most of them work. Other DMARDs are also categorized as *immunosuppressants*. This group includes methotrexate, azathioprine, cyclophosphamide, and cyclosporine. We *think* we know how they work: immunosuppressants appear to change the course of RA by suppressing, or decreasing the activity of, the immune system. The last and newest group of DMARDs, the **biologic response modifiers** (**BRMs**) (Enbrel, Remicade, Humira, and Kineret) are discussed in detail in Chapter 14.

As we have seen, in RA parts of the immune system are overactive, so a drug that decreases that hyperactivity of the immune system is useful in controlling the disease. But to maintain health, a person must have a properly functioning immune system, since the immune system is designed to fight infection. For this reason, immunosuppressants must be prescribed with care. The immune system cannot be allowed to become suppressed to the point that it is unable to fight infection. Safe and effective treatment of RA with immunosuppressants requires close supervision by a physician experienced in their use, preferably a **rheumatologist.**

Nonimmunosuppressant DMARDs

Injectable gold: gold sodium thiomalate (Myochrysine); Aurothioglucose (Solganal)

Generic available: yes
Usual dose: weekly to monthly injections
Effective within: six weeks to six months

Gold was first used as a medicine in the early 1900s, to treat people with tuberculosis and other infections. Believing that RA was caused by tuberculosis, Dr. Jacques Forestier began injecting gold into RA patients in the late 1920s, with a degree of success. During the 1930s and early 1940s, doctors prescribed very high doses of gold and achieved excellent results, although with excessive side effects. Eventually the disadvantages were considered to outweigh the benefits, and gold therapy went through a phase of disfavor.

In the late 1940s gold therapy began a resurgence, after carefully designed studies proved that lower doses could be effective. Since then, gold injections have been administered to thousands of people, many of whom have enjoyed positive results with few side effects. Although some rheumatologists consider gold to be an excellent therapy, many respected physicians question its usefulness, given the availability of newer DMARDs.

The two most commonly prescribed forms of injectable gold are approximately half gold by weight (and half inactive ingredients). The injections are administered into the buttock muscles. The dose is increased slowly over weeks and months, to limit side effects. Once improvement is noted, the interval between injections can be prolonged, although injections are generally not spaced further apart than one month. This frequency is usually necessary to sustain a remission.

Side effects of injectable gold. About one in every three persons receiving injectable gold will experience side effects from it (Table 7), skin rash and mouth sores being the most common problems. Approximately 15 percent of people treated will discontinue gold within the first six months because of its toxicity.

The kidneys are sometimes affected by gold therapy, although fewer

Table 7
Side Effects of Injectable Gold

Side Effects	Incidence	Side Effect Therapy
Nuisance		
Rash or itching	15–25%	Discontinue medication or reduce dosage; apply corticosteroid cream; take antihistamines
Mouth sores	5–10%	Discontinue medication if sores are severe or intolerable
Metallic taste		No treatment
Hair thinning (mild)		No treatment
Serious		
Blood toxicities	1–5%	Discontinue medication
Protein in urine	10–20% (significant in only 1–3%)	Discontinue medication if significant amounts of protein are present
Lung toxicity	Rare	Discontinue medication
Neuropathy	Rare	Discontinue medication
Colitis	Rare	Discontinue medication
Liver problems	Rare	Discontinue medication
Nitritoid reaction	5%	Discontinue medication or use aurothiogluclose (Solganal) instead of gold sodium thiomalate (Myochrysine)

than 1 percent of people receiving the treatments develop *serious* kidney problems. The most common problem is the appearance of protein in the urine. The vast majority of kidney problems reverse themselves when gold injections are discontinued.

Gold-induced blood problems are also rare. In 1 to 3 percent of patients, a low platelet count develops. This is almost always treatable and reversible. In fewer than 0.5 percent of people, serious bone marrow problems occur. Since the bone marrow produces red and white blood cells as well as platelets, this complication must be detected as early as possible and gold therapy discontinued. Everyone receiving gold injections must have their blood monitored closely and frequently. Early detection of a blood problem permits prompt treatment and usually reverses the problem.

Nitritoid reaction is an alarming but usually not dangerous occasional side effect. When it occurs, it happens within ten minutes after the injection has been given. Flushing, fainting, dizziness, and sweating are its symptoms. Although these symptoms can be frightening, they generally have no serious consequences. Fewer than 5 percent of people taking gold sodium thiomalate (Myochrysine) have this reaction. If this occurs the gold preparation can be changed to aurothioglucose (Solganal). Availability of both preparations has been a recent problem.

Before starting injectable gold therapy, discuss the following with your physician:

· A history of blood disorders, kidney or liver disease, uncontrolled high blood pressure, bleeding problems, or allergic reactions to any drugs

While receiving injectable gold:

· Contact your physician promptly if you notice a new rash or itching, mouth sores, increased bruising, a tendency to bleed easily, fever, cough, shortness of breath, or a change in skin or urine color.
· Avoid unprotected or prolonged exposure to the sun.
· Your doctor will frequently order tests for complete blood counts and urine studies.

Pregnancy and breastfeeding. Gold should probably be stopped several months before conception if possible. Gold is excreted in breast milk, and the potential exists for serious adverse effects in the nursing infant. Mothers should discontinue either nursing or gold injections.

Oral gold: Auranofin (Ridaura)

Generic available: no
Capsule size: 3 mg
Usual dose: one pill twice daily
Effective within: six weeks to six months

The introduction of auranofin in the 1980s allowed people with RA to take gold by mouth. This method of treatment can be effective in slowing the progression of RA, particularly if begun in the early stages of disease. Unlike injectable gold, oral gold is only 29 percent gold by weight. Many physicians believe that auranofin is not as effective as injectable gold.

Side effects of oral gold. Auranofin therapy results in fewer *serious* side effects than does injectable gold (Table 8). The most common side effects

Table 8
Side Effects of Oral Gold

Side Effects	Incidence	Side Effect Therapy
Nuisance		
Rash	24%	Discontinue medication or
Itching	17%	reduce dosage; apply corticosteroid cream
Hives	1–3%	Discontinue medication
Mouth sores	13%	Discontinue medication if sores are severe or intolerable
Diarrhea, abdominal cramps, decreased appetite, heartburn, flatulence	40–50%	Take medication with meals, take fiber laxatives, or increase dose slowly
Metallic taste	Rare	No treatment
Hair loss (minor)	2.4%	No treatment
Serious		
Blood problems	1–2%	Discontinue medication
Kidney problems	Less than 5%	Discontinue medication
Lung problems	Rare	Discontinue medication
Liver abnormalities	Rare	Discontinue medication

are stomach cramping, diarrhea, nausea, and changes in appetite. Most of these problems can be made tolerable by starting with a low dose, taking the medication with meals and consuming products containing bulk and large amounts of fiber, such as Metamucil and Fiberall.

Before starting auranofin therapy discuss the following with your physician:

· Previous history of blood disorders, kidney or liver disease, uncontrolled high blood pressure, bleeding problems, or allergic reactions to any drugs

While receiving auranofin:

· Contact your physician promptly if you notice a rash or itching, mouth sores, increased bruising, an increased tendency to bleed, fever, cough, shortness of breath, or a change in skin or urine color.
· Avoid unprotected or prolonged exposure to the sun.
· Complete blood counts and urine studies need to be done frequently during therapy.

Pregnancy and breastfeeding. Discontinue gold therapy during pregnancy. Gold is excreted in breast milk, and the potential exists for serious adverse effects in the nursing infant. Mothers should discontinue either nursing or auranofin therapy.

Hydroxychloroquine (Plaquenil)

Generic available: yes
Tablet size: 200 mg
Usual dose: one or two pills daily
Effective within: six weeks to six months

The healing qualities of quinine have been recognized for centuries. Quinine and its derivatives have been used to treat skin ailments, fever, and, notably, malaria. Commonly used antimalarial drugs are hydroxychloroquine, chloroquine, and quinacrine. Quinacrine was the first antimalarial medication used to treat RA. Its application to this purpose began in the 1950s. Chloroquine and hydroxychloroquine are both used today in treating RA. Hydroxychloroquine is used most commonly because it causes fewer side effects and is more available.

Side effects of hydroxychloroquine. Hydroxychloroquine may be the safest of all the DMARDs. Estimates are that only 5 percent of patients discontinue using the medication because of its side effects. The most commonly reported side effects of hydroxychloroquine are nausea, decreased appetite, diarrhea, and rash (Table 9). Most of these problems can be eliminated with dose changes and by taking the medication at mealtime.

The principal concern with all antimalarial drugs is the risk of eye problems (*retinopathy*). With long-term use, these medications can cause changes in the eye's retina. When hydroxycloroquine is taken in the customary dose for RA, however, the risk of this is exceedingly small. Dr. Howard Bernstein of Bethesda, Maryland, reports that the risk of retinopathy for patients taking 400 mg per day of hydroxycloroquine is less than 0.5 percent. When eye examinations are performed by an **ophthalmologist** every six months and the medication is discontinued immediately on the ophthalmologist's advice, the risk of permanent eye damage approaches 0 percent. Chloroquine use involves a slightly higher risk of permanent eye damage.

Your ophthalmologist may also mention that he or she has detected deposits on the cornea. This appears to be a reversible side effect that does not warrant a change in therapy.

When hydroxychloroquine is first taken, your vision may be tem-

Table 9
Side Effects of Hydroxychloroquine

Side Effects	Incidence	Side Effect Therapy
Nuisance		
Nausea, decreased appetite, diarrhea, bloating	11–20%	Take medication with meals or divide dosage
Rash	Occasional	Reduce dosage and apply corticosteroid cream
Skin pigment changes	10–25%	Discontinue medication if significant
Nervousness, headache, dizziness	Infrequent	Discontinue medication or reduce dosage
Serious		
Blood abnormalities	Rare	Discontinue medication
Eye problems		
Retinal damage	Rare	Discontinue medication
Corneal deposits	18–46%	Continue medication
Muscular weakness	Rare	Discontinue medication

porarily blurred. This does not mean that there is a problem with your retina; the blurring will clear within a week.

Before starting hydroxychloroquine therapy, discuss the following with your physician:

· A history of psoriasis, liver disease, porphyria, or eye problems
· Any medications that you are presently taking, particularly the heart medication digoxin
· If you have been diagnosed as having glucose-6-phosphate dehydrogenase (G-6-PD) deficiency. This condition appears in approximately 10 percent of black people and in some people of Mediterranean background. A blood test for G-6-PD deficiency can be performed before you start treatment with hydroxychloroquine.
· A baseline examination (an examination performed before treatment begins) by an ophthalmologist is recommended.

While taking hydroxychloroquine:

· Contact your physician promptly if you notice a change in vision, a rash, muscle weakness, fever, or easy bleeding or bruising.

· Avoid unprotected or prolonged exposure to the sun.
· You should be checked by an ophthalmologist every six months while taking this medication. (The manufacturer of Plaquenil recommends an ophthalmologic examination every three months.)

Pregnancy and breastfeeding. Because the eyes of the fetus can (rarely) be affected by hydroxychloroquine, it is recommended that use of this medication be avoided during pregnancy. Hydroxychloroquine is excreted in breast milk, and therefore mothers should discontinue either nursing or use of the medication.

Penicillamine (Cuprimine, Depen)

Generic available: no
Cuprimine capsule size: 125, 250 mg
Depen (scored) tablet size: 250 mg
Usual dose: two to four pills daily
Effective within: two to nine months

Penicillamine has been used since the 1960s to treat people with RA, and it is quite effective. It takes a long time to become effective, because its dose has to be increased very slowly to minimize side effects. This DMARD is infrequently used today, because there are now safer medications.

The chemical structure of penicillamine is similar to that of penicillin. Nevertheless, there seems to be no increased incidence of allergic reactions to this drug in individuals who are allergic to penicillin.

Side effects of penicillamine. Penicillamine therapy produces numerous side effects, which limits its use (Table 10). Withdrawal rates of up to 40 percent in the first year have been reported. Some of the serious side effects are similar to those of injectable gold. A chief concern is the development of blood abnormalities, the most common being decreased platelet counts, a condition that is usually reversible (approximately 4 percent of people taking penicillamine develop this condition). The white blood cell count decreases in approximately 2 percent of individuals using this drug. Low white blood cell counts are usually reversible, but the risk of infection is increased while the counts are low.

Kidney problems can develop with penicillamine treatment. Almost all of these problems can be reversed if they are detected early. Penicillamine therapy also can, rarely, result in the development of autoimmune conditions such as myasthenia gravis, pemphigus, Goodpasture's syndrome, or systemic lupus erythematosus. All of these conditions are serious but can be treated successfully.

Table 10
Side Effects of Penicillamine

Side Effects	Incidence	Side Effect Therapy
Nuisance		
Rash	12–25%	Discontinue medication or reduce dosage; take antihistamines
Upset stomach, nausea, vomiting, anorexia, diarrhea	12–20%	Reduce dosage
Change in taste	4–33%	Discontinue medication or reduce dosage
Breast enlargement	Rare	Continue medication
Mouth sores	10%	Reduce dosage
Serious		
Blood toxicities	5–10%	Discontinue medication
Protein in urine	6–20%	Discontinue medication or reduce dosage
Autoimmune syndromes	2%	Discontinue medication
Liver test abnormalities	Rare	Discontinue medication
Lung problems	Rare	Discontinue medication
Muscle weakness	1–2%	Discontinue medication

Before starting penicillamine therapy, discuss the following with your physician:

· A diagnosis of lupus
· A history of lung conditions, skin conditions, or kidney or liver disease

While taking penicillamine:

· Contact your physician promptly if you notice a new rash or itching, mouth sores, increased bruising, easy bleeding, fever, sore throat, cough, shortness of breath, or a change in urine or skin color.
· Take medication on an empty stomach (at least one hour before or two hours after a meal).
· Complete blood counts and urine studies need to be performed frequently during therapy.

Pregnancy and breastfeeding. Since penicillamine can cause birth defects, this medication is not to be taken during pregnancy. Nursing mothers should not take this medication.

Sulfasalazine (Azulfidine)

Generic available: yes
Tablet size: 500 mg
Enteric-coated tablets: 500 mg
Liquid form is available.
Usual dose: two or three pills twice daily
Effective within: two to six months

Sulfasalazine is commonly prescribed to treat colitis, although when it was developed in the 1930s by Professor Nanna Svartz in Stockholm it was designed for the treatment of RA. Sulfa drugs were just being developed at that time, and RA was considered to be an infectious condition. Sulfasalazine contained both an antibiotic (sulfa) and an anti-inflammatory component (salicylate). It was used to treat RA throughout the 1940s, with proven effectiveness, but eventually fell into disfavor for political reasons and because the new miracle drug, cortisone, had become available.

Since the late 1980s, there has been a resurgence of interest in and use of sulfasalazine for RA. This drug did not receive formal FDA approval for use in RA until 1996. Studies have determined that sulfasalazine can be used effectively alone or in combination with other DMARDs, such as methotrexate. Many rheumatologists prescribe sulfasalazine for RA because of its effectiveness and low incidence of serious side effects.

Side effects of sulfasalazine. Individuals taking this medication complain more frequently of stomach problems than of any other side effect (Table 11). Although sulfasalazine is most effective when taken on an empty stomach, taking it with meals is acceptable and helps prevent stomach discomfort. Enteric-coated tablets (available at a higher price than uncoated tablets) also help in this regard. Beginning treatment with low doses and increasing the dose slowly also improve stomach acceptance.

Decreased sperm counts and changes in the sperm can occur, temporarily decreasing fertility. Sperm counts return to normal approximately two months after sulfasalazine use has been discontinued.

Serious side effects are quite rare and usually appear early in the course of treatment. Most worrisome are severe sulfa allergic reactions, hepatitis, fever, and a decrease in the number of white blood cells, red blood cells, and platelets. The majority of people recover from these side effects when the medication is discontinued and proper treatment is given.

Table 11
Side Effects of Sulfasalazine

Side Effects	Incidence	Side Effect Therapy
Nuisance		
Nausea, vomiting, upset stomach	Greater than 20%	Take medication with meals; take enteric-coated tablets
Headache, irritability, dizziness	Less than 5%	Discontinue medication or reduce dosage
Rash	1–5%	Discontinue medication
Reduced sperm count		Discontinue medication
Serious		
Blood problems	0.5–4.0%	Discontinue medication
Liver toxicity	Rare	Discontinue medication
Allergic reaction	Common if sulfa allergic	Discontinue medication

Before starting sulfasalazine therapy, discuss the following with your physician:

· Allergy to sulfa or other antibiotics; allergy to aspirin or history of nasal polyps or bronchial asthma
· A history of kidney or liver problems
· Any medications you are taking to treat diabetes, blood pressure, seizures, or heart ailments or to thin the blood

While taking sulfasalazine:

· Avoid or protect yourself against sun exposure.
· Inform your physician immediately if you develop a rash, blood in your urine, fever, bruising or easy bleeding, sore throat, cough, or shortness of breath.
· Your physician will intermittently order complete blood counts, liver function tests, and urine tests to monitor and control the side effects.

Pregnancy and breastfeeding. Avoid use of this medication during pregnancy. Although birth defects have not been reported, caution suggests the use of birth control methods until sulfasalazine has been discontinued for two months.

Leflunamide (Arava)

Generic available: no
Tablet size: 100 mg (first three days only); 10, 20 mg
Usual dose: 100 mg tablet for first three days (loading dose), then one
   20 mg tablet daily; daily dose can be decreased to 10 mg if side
   effects appear
Effective within: one to three months

In late 1998, a new DMARD, leflunamide (Arava), became available. Unlike many of its predecessors, leflunamide was developed specifically to treat rheumatoid arthritis. Like other DMARDs, leflunamide helps to reduce joint swelling as well as slow the progression of joint damage. It appears to work differently than other available medications because it affects a unique stage in the process of RA. It is an immune system modifier which interferes with the proliferation (multiplication) of activated lymphocytes. (See sections on inflammation in Chapter 1.)

Studies suggest that leflunamide is an effective DMARD, comparable to methotrexate and sulfasalazine in effectiveness. Leflunamide is approved by the FDA for "slowing structural damage." Studies have also shown that leflunamide reduced tenderness and swelling in joints, and patients reported reduced pain levels and less difficulty performing activities of daily living, such as walking and dressing.

Side effects of leflunamide. The most commonly reported side effects associated with leflunamide are diarrhea and other gastrointestinal symptoms, such as bloating, nausea, and abdominal pain (Table 12). These problems are usually mild and short-lived. Some patients experience more serious symptoms, requiring a reduction of dosage or discontinuation of medication. Other side effects include skin rash, reversible hair loss, and elevations of liver enzymes. Cases of severe liver problems have been reported but are rare. (These cases have mostly occurred within the first six months of treatment. Many of these patients had other serious conditions or were on other medications that could be toxic to the liver.)

Leflunamide should be used with caution if you are taking other medications that can affect the liver. It should be avoided by people with a history of heavy alcohol use, hepatitis, or other severe liver problems. Laboratory tests, including liver function tests and complete blood counts, should be checked frequently during the first six months of treatment, then intermittently thereafter.

Before starting leflunamide therapy, discuss the following with your physician:

· The form of contraception you are using to avoid pregnancy

Table 12
Side Effects of Leflunamide

Side Effects	Incidence	Side Effect Therapy
Nuisance		
Diarrhea	17–27%	Usually goes away; if not, discontinue or reduce dosage
Nausea, vomiting, abdominal pain, decreased appetite	3–9%	Take medication with meals; discontinue or reduce dosage
Headache, dizziness, numbness	2–7%	Discontinue or reduce dosage
Hair loss	9–10%	Discontinue or reduce dosage
Rash	4–10%	Discontinue or reduce dosage
Serious		
Serious infection	Rare	Treat infection; discontinue medication until infection better
Liver problems	—	Reduce dosage and eliminate alcohol; possibly discontinue medication
Severe allergic reaction	Rare	Discontinue medication and consider drug elimination procedure with cholestyramine

· Any medications you are currently taking but in particular, rifampin or cholestyramine
· Any history of kidney or liver problems
· Present or past history of excessive alcohol use
· Any history of serious immune deficiency or uncontrolled infections

While taking leflunamide:

· Call your doctor if the onset of menstruation is delayed or you suspect pregnancy.
· Contact your physician with any signs of yellowing of your skin or eyes, or if there is a change in the color of your urine or stool.
· Avoid drinking alcohol.
· Inform your doctor if you develop signs of infection such as fever, chills, cough, burning with urination, or sore throat.
· Contact your physician if you develop a rash, shortness of breath, blood in your urine, or easy bruising.

- You may experience diarrhea; contact your doctor if the diarrhea is severe or does not diminish after the first two weeks of treatment.
- Your physician will initially order frequent laboratory tests to rule out potential side effects; in particular, complete blood counts and liver function tests should be monitored. If initial testing is unremarkable, further testing will be intermittent.
- If you miss a dose, do not double your dose the next day; just take routine dose.

Pregnancy, breastfeeding, and fatherhood. Animal testing indicates that leflunamide may result in birth defects if taken by a pregnant woman. Please be certain that you are not pregnant before starting this medication. Your physician may request a pregnancy test for you, to be certain. Reliable birth control measures are imperative while a woman is taking leflunamide. If you wish to become pregnant, a drug elimination procedure is required to remove leflunamide from your body. This is accomplished with the use of a medication called cholestyramine. This medication is given for 11 days, and then the blood is tested to confirm that leflunamide has been successfully eliminated. The test will then be repeated in another 14 days to be 100 percent certain of complete removal. Without cholestyramine, it takes *up to two years* for the body to remove leflunamide.

If you suspect you are pregnant, stop leflunamide immediately and contact your doctor for a pregnancy test. If you are pregnant, a drug elimination procedure is recommended with the use of cholestyramine. Further counseling from your obstetrician is then recommended. Arava should not be used by nursing mothers.

Although studies on men are limited, men are encouraged to stop treatment with leflunamide if considering a child. A drug elimination procedure with cholestyramine is suggested before attempting insemination.

Minocycline (Minocin)

Generic available: yes
Capsule size: 50, 100 mg
Usual dose: 100 mg twice daily
Effective within: two to four months

Minocycline is an antibiotic in the tetracycline family. Its story as it relates to RA is a very interesting one. For over fifty years, researchers have been trying to prove that there is an infectious cause or "trigger" for RA. One physician, Thomas McPherson Brown, ardently believed this to be true. Just before World War II, this young researcher isolated a microorganism, mycoplasma, from the joint fluid of a woman with RA. This finding could not be confirmed by other researchers, and so it was discounted by the scientific world. Despite this, Dr. Brown started treating patients with tetracycline-type antibiotics and had good results. He published a report on 98 of his patients in 1985; because his study was not a "double-blind" study, his results were not considered scientifically valid. Dr. Brown wrote a widely circulated book called *The Road Back* describing his unique perspective as an early pioneer in this area (Brown's work included in Scammell, 1998).

In the last decade, several scientific studies have shown that minocycline *is* a safe and effective treatment for RA. The largest of these trials, called the MIRA trial (minocycline in rheumatoid arthritis) was published in 1995 (Tilley et al., 1995). After this report, many physicians began prescribing minocycline for RA. Researchers are not certain whether the antibiotic effect of minocycline is what renders it effective for RA. The tetracycline family of antibiotics appears to have other effects on the immune system and inflammatory proteins that may play a role. There are strong proponents of the "microorganism theory" and the "immunomodulatory theory" for its effectiveness. Minocycline has not been approved by the FDA for use in RA and likely will never be. The studies needed for FDA approval are very costly, and since this medication is available in a generic form, there is no source of funding to perform the necessary testing required for approval. The drug has been approved for long-term treatment of acne and should not be considered experimental for that purpose. Because of its widespread use, effectiveness, and safety, this medication has become a commonly prescribed DMARD, particularly in patients with mild, early RA.

Side effects of minocycline. Minocycline has very few side effects compared to other DMARDs (Table 13). The most common complaint is dizziness. In most cases this is mild, but it can be significant enough to make some patients discontinue use. Other potential side effects are rash and stomach problems. Infrequently, some patients describe changes in skin pigmentation. Rarely, a bluish discoloration can occur on the skin and inside the mouth. Although the rash is not harmful, most individuals choose to discontinue the medication if it occurs. Like other antibiotics, minocycline can cause overgrowth of fungi or yeast in some patients. This is more likely to occur if someone has had a previous history of yeast or *Candida* infections. Increased sensitivity to the sun is a possibility, so persons taking minocycline need to be cautious about intense sun exposure. Rarely, this medication has been associated with the development of lupus-like symptoms.

Before starting minocycline therapy, discuss the following with your physician:

Table 13
Side Effects of Minocycline

Side Effects	Incidence	Side Effect Therapy
Nuisance		
Rash	Infrequent	Discontinue medication
Photosensitivity	Occasional	Avoid intense sun; use sun protection
Pigmentation of skin and mucous membranes	Rare	Discontinue medication if significant
Lightheadedness, dizziness or vertigo	Occasional	Contact your physician; often self-limiting; may need to discontinue medication
Nausea, diarrhea, decreased appetite	Infrequent	Discontinue if significant
Yeast or *Candida* infections	Infrequent	Treat yeast infection; may need to discontinue if severe or recurrent infection
Serious		
Severe dizziness and headache	Rare	Discontinue medication
Abnormal liver tests; hepatitis	Rare	Discontinue medication
Severe allergic reaction	Rare	Discontinue medication
Decreased hearing	Rare	Discontinue medication
Blood abnormalities	Rare	Discontinue medication
Lupus-like condition	Rare	Discontinue medication

· Any side effects that you have had with antibiotics, particularly the tetracycline family of antibiotics
· Use of birth control pills, because minocycline may make oral contraceptives less effective
· Use of warfarin or Coumadin; close observation and dosage adjustment may be required
· History of serious kidney or liver disease
· History of yeast infections

While taking minocycline:

· Contact your physician with any new or unusual symptoms.
· Avoid taking this medication at the same time as antacids, calcium,

magnesium, or iron, since they may interfere with absorption of minocycline.
· Be careful to avoid high-intensity sun exposure and tanning beds; use
sun blockers and protective clothing.
· If you experience dizziness while on minocycline, avoid driving vehicles
or using hazardous machinery; contact your physician if dizziness is
severe.
· Temporarily stop minocycline if you are on another antibiotic for an
infection, since the antibiotics may compete with each other.

Pregnancy and breastfeeding. Minocycline can cause fetal harm when
taken by a pregnant woman. The use of minocycline during fetal tooth
development (latter half of pregnancy) may cause permanent discoloration of the teeth. Minocycline is excreted in breast milk. Nursing infants
would be at risk for permanent tooth discoloration.

Immunosuppressants

Methotrexate (Rheumatrex)

Generic available: yes
Tablet size: 2.5 mg
Usual dose: two to eight pills per week all on one day, or in one weekly
   injection
Effective within: three to eight weeks

Methotrexate was used initially in the 1940s to treat people with leukemia
and is still frequently taken in very high doses as an anticancer drug. It
later became widely used as a treatment for severe psoriasis and a form
of arthritis associated with this skin condition. Since the early 1980s its
use in the treatment of RA has skyrocketed, and it is now the most commonly prescribed DMARD.
   The marked increase in this drug's popularity for RA treatment has
many explanations. First, it becomes effective more rapidly than the traditional DMARDs: improvement is sometimes noted within two weeks of
the first use. Second, it is very effective. Third, it is very convenient in that
it can be taken once a week.

Side effects of methotrexate. Like the other immunosuppressants, methotrexate can produce side effects (Table 14). The most commonly reported
ones involve stomach and mouth sores. Nausea, vomiting, and diarrhea
can usually be minimized by dividing up the weekly dose; that is, someone who experiences stomach problems from methotrexate can take the

Table 14
Side Effects of Methotrexate

Side Effects	Incidence	Side Effect Therapy
Nuisance		
Rash	1–11%	Discontinue medication or reduce dosage
Stomach problems		
Nausea	10–23%	Take medication with meals,
Vomiting	4%	adjust dosage, or take nausea medication
Diarrhea	8%	Take medication with meals
Mouth sores	3–10%	Reduce dosage or take folate or folinic acid
Headache	9%	Reduce dosage
Hair loss or thinning	1–5%	Reduce dosage
Dizziness	2%	Reduce dosage
Increase in nodules	Unknown	No treatment
Serious		
Liver problems	15%	Reduce dosage, eliminate alcohol, and reduce weight; possibly discontinue medication
Blood problems	1–10%	Reduce dosage or discontinue medication
Lung inflammation	2–5.5%	Discontinue medication and take corticosteroids
Stomach ulcers	Rare	Discontinue medication and take stomach medication
Infection	3.8%	Treat infection and discontinue medication

weekly dose of pills one pill every several hours (if your dose is three pills per week, for example, you would take one pill every eight hours on the day of your treatment). You cannot divide the dose up throughout the week, however. Your doctor will help you with a schedule that is tolerable for you. Other possibilities include taking the medication with food, adjusting the dose, and taking antinausea medications. Some people tolerate an intramuscular shot of methotrexate better than the pill form. Also, some physicians allow their patients to self-administer shots of methotrexate at home, if that person can demonstrate proper and safe technique. Home injections are usually given subcutaneously ("sub Q") or just under the skin.

The most frequent side effect that causes concern involves the liver. In people taking methotrexate, blood tests that measure liver enzymes are frequently elevated slightly, but this is rarely an indication of a serious liver problem. With long-term use, however, inflammation and scarring of the liver can take place. Although cirrhosis of the liver is a distinctly rare side effect, some people with psoriatic arthritis have developed cirrhosis of the liver from methotrexate. Scarring and cirrhosis appear to be much less common in RA patients. The risk of liver problems can be minimized greatly if the person avoids alcohol and keeps his or her weight down. After several years of methotrexate use, a liver biopsy may be indicated, particularly if liver function test abnormalities appear and persist.

Blood counts (white and red blood cells and platelets) can be lowered by methotrexate use. At the dose used to treat RA, this side effect is unusual. When it occurs, it is almost always reversible by discontinuing the use or reducing the dose of the drug. Reduced platelet counts increase bleeding risks in some people. When the white blood cell count is markedly lowered, serious infections can occur; much more rarely, unusual, or atypical, infections develop while white blood counts are at *normal* levels. These infections can develop because of methotrexate's effect on the immune system.

Another serious side effect is lung inflammation, or pneumonitis. This inflammation is generally reversible with discontinuation of methotrexate and treatment with **corticosteroids.** Pneumonitis can, on rare occasions, be life threatening. Smoking appears to increase the risk.

Recent studies suggest that taking folic acid (or folate) supplements decreases the side effects of methotrexate. Some physicians also prescribe folinic acid before each methotrexate dose if side effects are significant.

Before starting methotrexate therapy, discuss the following with your physician:

· A history of liver problems (especially hepatitis), stomach ulcer, alcohol use, kidney or lung problems, blood problems, human immunodeficiency virus (HIV) infection, or a positive tuberculin skin test or tuberculosis
· Any medications you are currently taking, but particularly sulfa drugs, other antibiotics (particularly those containing trimethaprim), NSAIDs, diuretics (water pills), probenecid (gout medication), and medications to treat seizures or diabetes

While taking methotrexate:

· Contact your physician promptly if you have mouth sores, nausea or vomiting, black or tar-colored stools, fever or chills, sore throat, unusual bleeding or bruising, a change in skin or urine color, cough or shortness of breath, or a marked increase in fatigue.
· Inform your doctor if you have an infection; methotrexate is often temporarily discontinued to help your immune system fight infection.
· Inform your physician, surgeon, or dentist that you are taking methotrexate *well before* he or she performs any medical procedure.
· Ask your physician before you receive any "live" vaccines; flu and pneumonia vaccinations are generally recommended.
· *Never* take this medication more than one day a week.
· Alcohol ingestion is prohibited.
· Take *every* precaution to avoid pregnancy (see below).
· Frequent liver function tests and blood tests to obtain complete blood counts are required. Blood tests for kidney function and urine studies may be requested periodically by your physician.

Pregnancy and breastfeeding. Methotrexate is an extremely dangerous medication for the fetus. It has been known to cause fetal death and birth defects. Women should avoid getting pregnant for *at least* one full menstrual cycle after stopping methotrexate. Men should wait *at least* three months after discontinuing methotrexate treatment before trying to father children. Do not breastfeed while taking methotrexate.

Azathioprine (Imuran)

Generic available: yes
Tablet size: 50 mg
Usual dose: variable
Effective within: six weeks to six months

Azathioprine was initially introduced as a form of cancer chemotherapy and is still being used for that purpose. It is also used to prevent rejection in organ transplant recipients. It was the first immunosuppressant to be approved by the FDA for use in RA and has been shown to be an effective treatment. Many physicians prefer to reserve this therapy for patients who have not responded to treatment with other DMARDs. Azathioprine is a notable component in many combination therapies.

Side effects of azathioprine. The side effect of most concern with azathioprine use is blood abnormalities, most commonly a lowered white blood cell count (Table 15). Infection can result and can become severe

Table 15
Side Effects of Azathioprine

Side Effects	Incidence	Side Effect Therapy
Nuisance		
Nausea, vomiting, diarrhea	12–16%	Take medication with meals or divide dosage
Rash	2%	Discontinue medication or reduce dosage
Mouth sores	Rare	Reduce dosage
Hair loss	Rare	Reduce dosage or discontinue medication
Serious		
Infection	1–3%	Take antibiotics and discontinue medication
Liver problems	Rare	Discontinue medication
Blood problems	28%	Reduce dosage or discontinue medication
Cancer risks	(See text)	
Pancreatitis	Rare	Discontinue medication

when insufficient numbers of white blood cells are present to destroy infection-causing bacteria. As with other immunosuppressants, there is also an increased risk of unusual infections even without a change in the white blood cell count. Less common blood abnormalities include decreased numbers of platelets or red blood cells (resulting in **anemia**). With low numbers of platelets, bruising or bleeding may occur more easily. Blood abnormalities almost always improve when azathioprine is discontinued. Life-threatening situations are rare. Any person taking azathioprine *must* be monitored vigilantly by a physician who is an expert in immunosuppressant therapy.

Another side effect that has received a great deal of attention is the risk of developing cancer after prolonged use of azathioprine. This concern is debated in rheumatology circles. Findings from studies of large numbers of RA patients taking azathioprine in the United Kingdom are reassuring. These studies suggest that the additional risk of cancer, although it exists, in people taking azathioprine as compared with others with RA, is actually quite small.

Before starting azathioprine therapy, discuss the following with your physician:

· A history of blood problems, liver or kidney disease, HIV infection, or a positive tuberculin skin test or tuberculosis
· All medications that you are taking, but in particular allopurinol (gout medicine) and angiotensin converting enzyme (ACE) inhibitors (a blood pressure medicine)

While you are taking azathioprine:

· Contact your physician promptly if you notice fever or chills, sore throat, cough, unusual bruising or bleeding, a marked increase in fatigue, nausea or stomach pain, or a change in urine or skin color.
· Inform your doctor if you have an infection; azathioprine is often discontinued on a temporary basis to help your immune system combat the infection.
· Ask your doctor before you receive any "live" vaccines; flu and pneumonia vaccinations are generally recommended.
· Take your medication with meals.
· *Never* take a dose higher than the doctor has prescribed.
· Try to avoid close contact with anyone who has a bacterial or viral infection.
· Frequent blood tests for blood counts and liver function tests are required.

Pregnancy and breastfeeding. Because problems can develop in the fetal immune system when the mother takes azathioprine, this medication should not be used during pregnancy, nor should it be taken if the mother is nursing.

Cyclophosphamide (Cytoxan)

Generic available: yes
Tablet size: 25, 50 mg
Intravenous administration possible
Dose: variable
Effective within: two weeks to three months

Cyclophosphamide is by far the most potent and dangerous of the immunosuppressive drugs used in the treatment of RA. Like azathioprine, it was first used as a form of cancer chemotherapy. Its effectiveness in the treatment of RA is undisputed, but its potentially severe side effects preclude its use in the treatment of mild or moderate RA. Cyclophosphamide is generally reserved for the treatment of unusually severe or life-

Table 16
Side Effects of Cyclophosphamide

Side Effects	Incidence	Side Effect Therapy
Nuisance		
Nausea, vomiting, decreased appetite	Common	Take nausea medication
Rash	Less than 5%	Discontinue medication or reduce dosage
Hair loss	Common[a]	Reduce dosage if possible
Serious		
Blood problems	(See text)[a]	Discontinue medication or reduce dosage
Bladder problems	17%	Discontinue medication and drink ample fluid to facilitate frequent urination
Infection	(See text)[a]	Treat infection and discontinue medication if possible
Cancer risks	(See text)[a]	Treat cancer
Liver problems	Rare	Discontinue medication
Lung problems	Rare	Discontinue medication
Infertility	Common[a]	No treatment

[a] Frequency depends on dose and length of time medication is taken.

threatening complications of RA, such as **vasculitis, Felty's syndrome,** and other complications with organ involvement (see Chapter 4 for more about these). In these very serious situations, the benefits of cyclophosphamide outweigh the risks.

Side effects of cyclophosphamide. Cyclophosphamide has essentially the same potential side effects as azathioprine (see above and Table 16). Because cyclophosphamide has a more potent effect on the bone marrow and immune system, the occurrence and severity of these side effects are higher than in people taking azathioprine, although the precise risk is difficult to ascertain. We do know that a low white blood cell count occurs so frequently during cyclophosphamide therapy that it is often considered an *expected effect* rather than a side effect. The risk of severe blood abnormalities and infection increases in proportion to the dose and length of time which cyclophosphamide is prescribed.

Unlike azathioprine, cyclophosphamide can cause *cystitis* or bladder inflammation. Uncomfortable urination and the appearance of blood in the urine are symptoms of cystitis.

Hair loss can occur, particularly at very high doses. The amount of hair loss is highly variable, but in almost all patients it regrows after the treatment is discontinued.

An important concern in cyclophosphamide therapy is the long-term increased risk of bladder cancer or blood cancers (leukemias and lymphomas). It is estimated that with long-term daily cyclophosphamide use the risk of developing these cancers nearly doubles. Because cyclophosphamide is prescribed almost exclusively for severe, unremitting RA or for life-threatening complications, this potential risk of cancer in the future is usually at a tolerable level.

Before starting cyclophosphamide therapy, discuss the following with your physician:

· A history of blood problems, kidney or liver conditions, HIV infection, previous x-ray therapy or chemotherapy, or a positive tuberculin skin test or tuberculosis
· Any medications you are taking, but in particular sleeping medications (barbiturates), diuretics (water pills), or gout medications (allopurinol)

While taking cyclophosphamide:

· Contact your physician promptly if you notice fever or chills, sore throat, cough, unusual bleeding or bruising, a change in urine color, burning or pain with urination, a change in skin color, or a marked increase in fatigue.
· Contact your physician at any sign of infection; cyclophosphamide is often discontinued on a temporary basis to help your immune system combat infection.
· Ask your doctor before you receive any "live" vaccines; flu and pneumonia vaccinations are generally recommended.
· Monitor your urination while you are taking cyclophosphamide. Make certain that the frequency of urination has not decreased. Drink large amounts of water each day to flush out your bladder.
· Never take this medication at bedtime.
· Avoid close contact with anyone who has a viral or bacterial infection.

Pregnancy and breastfeeding. Both men and women must use contraception while taking cyclophosphamide. *Birth defects are a distinct possibility.* Decreased fertility and sterility are potential side effects of this medication. Nursing is not recommended.

Cyclosporine (Neoral, Sandimmune)

Generic available: no
Neoral capsule size: 25, 100 mg
Liquid form: oral solution 100 mg/ml
Usual dose: varies with weight; usually taken twice per day
Effective within: four to eight weeks

When a single DMARD is not effective, your physician may choose to begin combination therapy, using more than one medication. Cyclosporine plus methotrexate is a DMARD combination that has been recommended for patients with severe active RA that is not responding to methotrexate alone. This combination treatment for RA was approved by the FDA in the late 1990s. However, cyclosporine had been used to treat RA for many years before then in countries other than the United States.

Cyclosporine is a powerful immunosuppressant that has been approved for use in the United States since the early 1980s for people who have undergone organ transplantation. Cyclosporine helps keep the immune system from rejecting the newly transplanted organ.

Because of its effect on the immune system, cyclosporine has also been shown to benefit patients with RA. Although sometimes prescribed alone, cyclosporine is most commonly prescribed with methotrexate. The FDA has not approved its use singly as a DMARD. In research studies, patients with severe rheumatoid arthritis who had partially responded to methotrexate alone had meaningful improvement with the combination of methotrexate and cyclosporine. These patients experienced less tenderness and swelling in their joints. Also, pain and degree of disability were reduced. Because of potential side effects, the patient should be placed on the lowest effective dose. If adverse effects do occur, the dose should be further reduced. Cyclosporine should be discontinued if there is no benefit at 16 weeks or if dose reduction does not eliminate side effects.

Side effects of cyclosporine. Side effects that may occur with the use of cyclosporine include high blood pressure and kidney problems (Table 17). The physician will likely check blood pressure and order kidney function tests frequently when a patient is starting with this medication. In clinical research trials, cyclosporine had to be discontinued in 5.3 percent of patients because of high blood pressure and in 7 percent of patients because of abnormal kidney tests (elevated creatinine). These serious side effects usually resolve after discontinuing the medication. Other potential problems include headache, stomach intolerance, and abnormal hair growth. As with other immunosuppressants, patients must be watched closely for

Table 17
Side Effects of Cyclosporine

Side Effects	Incidence	Side Effect Therapy
Nuisance		
Tremor	7–13%	Reduce dosage or discontinue medication
Headache	17–25%	Reduce dosage or discontinue medication
Dizziness	6–8%	Reduce dosage or discontinue medication
Burning or tingling sensations	7–11%	Reduce dosage or discontinue medication
Rash	7–12%	Reduce dosage or discontinue medication
Increased body hair	15–19%	Reduce dosage or discontinue medication
Nausea, diarrhea, upset stomach	15–24%	Reduce dosage or discontinue medication
Leg cramps	2–12%	Reduce dosage or discontinue medication
Reduced kidney function (by >30%)	39–48%	Reduce dosage or discontinue medication
Serious		
High blood pressure	8–26%	Reduce dosage or discontinue medication
Fluid retention	5–14%	Reduce dosage or discontinue medication
Reduced kidney function (by >50%)	18–24%	Reduce dosage or discontinue medication
Upper respiratory complications	3–14%	Reduce dosage or discontinue medication
Cancer (lymphoma)	Rare	Discontinue medication

possible infections. If you are on methotrexate as well, monthly blood counts and liver tests are also recommended in order to detect potential side effects early (see section on methotrexate). Only physicians experienced in management of immunosuppressive therapy for RA should prescribe cyclosporine and methotrexate in combination.

Before starting cyclosporine therapy, discuss the following with your physician:

· Any history of kidney problems or high blood pressure
· All current medications, because drug interactions are common
· Any history of immune deficiency or severe infections
· Any history of tuberculosis or a positive tuberculin skin test

While taking cyclosporine:

· Contact your doctor immediately with any signs of fever, chills, sinus pain, severe headache, cough, shortness of breath, pain or burning with urination, bleeding gums, or severe bruising.
· Contact your physician if you have an infection; he or she may want to discontinue the cyclosporine temporarily to help your immune system fight infection.
· You will need frequent monitoring of blood pressure, complete blood count, kidney function tests, and liver enzyme checks. Blood lipids, magnesium, potassium, and cyclosporine concentration may also require monitoring.
· Do *not* get any "live" vaccines; ask your doctor about any vaccines; flu and pneumonia vaccination are generally recommended.
· Alert your prescribing physician about *all* new medications (even over-the-counter ones) but, in particular, antibiotics, anti-inflammatory, stomach, blood pressure, heart, and seizure medications.

Pregnancy and breastfeeding. There are no adequate studies in pregnant women. Discontinuation of cyclosporine in non–life-threatening conditions is recommended. Cyclosporine is excreted in breast milk and should be avoided during breastfeeding.

For More Information

The makers of Arava (the brand name of leflunamide) have a toll-free information line and a Web site: 1-800-716-7168, www.rawatch.com.

CHAPTER 14

Biologic Response Modifiers (BRMs) and a Biologic Medical Device

•

Understanding Cytokines and Inflammation

Scientists are getting closer to understanding the very complex nature of rheumatoid arthritis. Researchers are discovering critical changes that occur in the immune system in people with RA. As these key elements are discovered, each piece of the puzzle gives us a new opportunity to target treatment. We use the word *target* because that is exactly what the newest class of medications does. These new treatments focus on a very small part of the complicated cascade of events that create and perpetuate RA. These new medications are called biologic response modifiers (BRMs) or, more commonly, *biologics*. Later in this chapter, we will review the BRMs that are currently available. Understanding this complex area is not easy, even for physicians. The following information is simply meant to give the reader an idea of the many revolutionary treatments that will be available in the future.

Biologic response modifiers use innovative tactics aimed at interfering with the cascade of events that lead to inflammation and damage. Before you can understand how the biologics work, it is important to understand some of the fundamental changes in the immune system that occur with rheumatoid inflammation. The normal immune system relies upon the communication between cells that is enabled by chemical messengers called *cytokines*. Cytokines communicate their message by attaching to *receptors* that are bound to the cells that are receiving the message. When the messenger (cytokine) connects to the receiving cell's receptor, the message is delivered. When a cytokine's message is "promote inflammation," the attachment of the cytokine to its receptor "turns on" the immune system cell (Figure 18). Once activated, the receiving cell releases chemicals that lead to inflammation and damage.

The two major cytokines that we know deliver the inflammation message are tumor necrosis factor (TNF) and interleukin-1 (IL-1). These mes-

Pro-inflammatory
cytokines

Inflammation

Pro-inflammatory
cytokine receptor

Immune cell
releasing
pro-inflammatory cytokine

Target immune cell
activated by
pro-inflammatory cytokine

Figure 18. Pro-inflammatory cytokines

sengers that promote inflammation are called pro-inflammatory cytokines. To balance them there are naturally occurring proteins that decrease inflammation by overpowering the pro-inflammatory messengers. The pro-inflammatory cytokines are not necessarily bad. They appear to have an important role in helping the immune system function properly. Pro-inflammatory cytokines, like TNF and IL-1, appear to have important *beneficial* functions in the body, but in RA their concentrations are abnormally high. *Completely* eliminating these pro-inflammatory cytokines is not the goal of treatment; putting them back in balance is.

Using the Body's Secrets to Tame Inflammation: Creating the Biologics

Naturally occurring anti-inflammatory proteins represent the body's built-in mechanism for balancing increased amounts of pro-inflammatory cytokines. One type of these proteins works by preventing the pro-inflammatory cytokine from hooking up to its receptor and delivering its message to the cell. These blocking agents are called *receptor antagonists*. They work by plugging up the receptor so it cannot receive the inflammation message delivered by the pro-inflammatory cytokine (Figure 19). We can mimic this type of anti-inflammatory protein with medication such as anakinra (Kineret). Kineret is a man-made receptor antagonist that plugs up the IL-1 receptor, preventing IL-1 from delivering its inflammation message. (It is specific to the IL-1 cytokine and does not affect TNF; TNF receptor antagonists are also being studied.)

The body also makes protective *free-floating receptors* that are not

Figure 19. Receptor antagonists

Figure 20. Soluble receptors

bound to cells. They can intercept the pro-inflammatory cytokines and knock them out of commission. These are called *soluble receptors* (Figure 20). These protective proteins naturally increase in the body in an effort to control inflammation. In essence, they snatch up the cytokine so it doesn't get to the target cell's receptor to deliver its inflammation message. We mimic this type of protein with a medication called etanercept (Enbrel). Enbrel is a biogenetically engineered soluble receptor that captures

Figure 21. Monoclonal antibodies

TNF before it can connect to its receptor and deliver its inflammation message. Soluble receptors for other pro-inflammatory cytokines are also being studied.

In addition to copying the body's built-in defenders of inflammation, technological agents can decrease the number of pro-inflammatory cytokines. One area of considerable research interest is the assembling of man-made antibodies called *monoclonal antibodies,* which are directed against the pro-inflammatory cytokines, rendering them inoperative (Figure 21). Monoclonal antibodies against TNF include infliximab (Remicade) and adalimumab (Humira). This technology for developing "man-made" antibodies against very specific targets seen several other medical applications and is a very exciting area of medical research.

Thus, our *current* biologic treatment options fall into two basic categories. The first strategy is to copy naturally occurring anti-inflammatory proteins, like receptor antagonists and soluble receptors, increasing their presence in the body in an effort to control inflammation, mimicking the natural response of the body to balance inflammation. The second strategy is to make monoclonal antibodies against the pro-inflammatory cytokine, reducing its effect in the body. Other antibody-like proteins are currently being studied. These "antibody fragments" can also be directed against pro-inflammatory cytokines. Some of the cytokine blockers just mentioned are described below (and see Table 18).

Table 18
Treatments to Reduce or Block Pro-inflammatory Cytokines

Pro-inflammatory Cytokine	Type of Potential Blocker	Availability
Tumor necrosis factor (TNF)		
	TNF soluble receptor	Enbrel (etanercept)—1998
	Monoclonal antibody against TNF	Remicade (infliximab)—November 1999
	Monoclonal antibody against TNF	Humira (adalimumab)—2003
	TNF soluble receptor	In research by Amgen
	Antibody fragment against TNF	In early research by Celltech
	Oral TNF binding protein	In early research by Amgen
	Oral TNF inhibitor	In early research by Scios
Interleukin-1 (IL-1)		
	IL-1 receptor antagonist	Kineret (anakinra)—2001
	IL-1 soluble receptor	In early research by Amgen
	IL-1 cytokine trap	In early research by Regeneron

Biologic Response Modifiers against TNF

Etanercept (Enbrel)

Generic available: no
Usual dose: 25 mg, by self-administered injection twice weekly
Effective within: two weeks to three months

Released in 1998, Enbrel was the first BRM available for the treatment of rheumatoid arthritis. Its introduction has forever changed the way we treat RA, giving patients and doctors an exciting and powerful way to manage the damaging effects of RA.

As mentioned above, cytokines, such as TNF, can increase inflammation. Although a small amount of TNF is necessary for the immune system to function normally, this cytokine is found in very high amounts in rheumatoid joints. High levels of TNF are believed to influence the pain, swelling, stiffness, and fatigue of rheumatoid arthritis. In the normal immune system, the body controls and balances the effects of TNF by producing a protein called soluble TNF receptor (see Figure 20). This protein captures or "mops up" TNF before it can connect to immune cells and cause inflammation.

Enbrel is a biologic drug in the category commonly called TNF blockers or anti-TNF drugs. This man-made (or "biotech") drug resembles the natural soluble TNF receptor. Enbrel, like its natural protein counterpart, binds to TNF. When bound to Enbrel, TNF cannot connect to cells and communicate its message to cause inflammation. Enbrel works *with* the naturally occurring protein to disarm the extra TNF that is produced in RA. Hence, Enbrel *adds to* the body's natural response to inflammation.

In medical studies, Enbrel has been shown to decrease pain, reduce tiredness, and decrease stiffness. Enbrel may provide relief as quickly as within two weeks; most people notice maximum benefits by three months. For many people, the positive effects of Enbrel are dramatic. In addition to reduced arthritis symptoms, they also report improvement in day to day functioning and vitality. Enbrel is used to treat moderately to severely active RA in people who have not adequately responded to traditional disease-modifying antirheumatic drugs (DMARDs), such as methotrexate. It may also be indicated as a first-line treatment in people with early RA who are deemed at high risk for rapidly progressive arthritis. Enbrel has been proven in clinical studies to delay structural damage and to slow the progression of arthritis.

Enbrel can be used alone as a *monotherapy*. If you are already on methotrexate and have had an inadequate result, Enbrel can be added as a form of *combination therapy*. In both cases, Enbrel has been proven to have remarkable results. Long-term studies are revealing that most patients have continued benefit.

Because Enbrel is a protein, it has to be injected by needle through the skin. If it were taken by mouth, it would be broken down by stomach enzymes and not be effective. The injection is given just beneath the skin. This is called a *subcutaneous* or *"sub Q"* injection. Many people are initially frightened or concerned about giving themselves a shot. Almost everyone, however, learns, under the guidance of their physician or nurse, to self-inject Enbrel without too much difficulty. The area of injection is "rotated" from site to site (thigh, abdomen, and arm) so no area gets too tender. It is best to have a friend or another person in the household learn to give injections. Then, if your hands are too sore, this care partner can help you. He or she can also inject areas that you cannot reach if that is needed. Of course, your physician and his or her staff will always be there if problems with self-administration develop.

Being a protein, Enbrel must also be refrigerated, at 36° to 46°F (although it must not freeze). If you are traveling, an insulated bag or cooler will be required to keep Enbrel at the correct temperature. A health professional will teach you how to reconstitute the concentrated solution provided by the pharmacy. If not administered immediately, the solution should be refrigerated and used within six hours. For safety, needles and syringes must be disposed of in a puncture-resistant container. Ask your doctor or nurse how you should dispose of the container in your community.

Because Enbrel is somewhat complicated to take correctly, unlike medications taken by mouth, the makers of Enbrel provide an educational program called Enliven, which provides newsletters, helpful hints, and a toll-free patient-support line. You should call your rheumatologist with any questions or concerns.

Enbrel is expensive, and your insurance company may require a "prior authorization," "precertification," or "letter of medical necessity" from your prescribing physician. If Enbrel is being considered, call your insurance company to inquire about their specific requirements.

Side effects of Enbrel. Fortunately, Enbrel has very few side effects for the vast majority of people (Table 19). The most common side effect is redness, itching, pain, or swelling at the injection site. These injection site reactions occur in just over one-third of people. They generally occur at the beginning of treatment, are usually mild, and resolve without specific treatment.

The most serious problem is increased risk of infection. Infections are mild in most circumstances. Here is what Enbrel's manufacturer says about other circumstances: "Since the product was first introduced, seri-

Table 19
Side Effects of Enbrel

Side Effects	Incidence	Side Effect Therapy
Nuisance		
Injection site reactions	37%	Review injection technique; observe closely
Headaches	17%	Discontinue if severe
Runny nose	12%	Monitor closely for infection
Nausea	9%	Treat symptoms
Serious		
Infection	32%	Discontinue; seek medical attention

ous infections, some involving death, have been reported in patients using Enbrel. Many of these events occurred in patients who were prone to infections, such as those with advanced or poorly controlled diabetes. Enbrel should be discontinued in patients with serious infections. Do not start Enbrel if you have an infection of any type or if you have an allergy to Enbrel or its components. Enbrel should be used with caution in patients prone to infection" (Enbrel package insert from Immunex [2001]). There have been cases of "reactivation" of tuberculosis in people who had been exposed to TB. If you have had a history of TB or have been exposed in the past, share that information with your physician before starting Enbrel.

Further cautions published by the manufacturer include these: "There have been rare reports of serious nervous system disorders such as multiple sclerosis and/or inflammation of the nerves of the eyes. Tell your doctor if you ever had any of these disorders or if you develop them after starting Enbrel. There have been rare reports of serious blood disorders, some involving death. Contact your doctor immediately if you develop symptoms such as persistent fever, bruising, bleeding, or paleness. It is unclear if Enbrel has caused these nervous system or blood disorders. If your doctor confirms serious blood problems, you may need to stop Enbrel" (package insert).

Before starting Enbrel therapy, discuss the following with your physician:

· Any poorly controlled diabetes, open wounds, signs of infection, predisposition to infection, history of tuberculosis or other serious infections
· The need for a TB skin test and/or a chest x-ray to see if there is evidence of previous tuberculosis
· If you have a latex allergy, since the needle cover contains latex

While receiving Enbrel:

· Contact your physician if you think that you are developing any kind of infection. Enbrel will be temporarily discontinued in most situations.
· If you experience severe redness, itching, pain, swelling, or any worrisome symptoms at an injection site, notify your doctor.
· Never inject into a tender, red, or hard area on the skin.
· Never inject Enbrel that has not been properly refrigerated.
· Do *not* get any "live" vaccines. Flu shots are a form of "killed" or inactivated vaccine and *should* be given in most circumstances. Pneumonia vaccinations are generally recommended.
· Contact your prescribing doctor if you are planning a surgery; many physicians choose to discontinue Enbrel temporarily around the time of the operation to reduce the risk of infection.

Pregnancy and breastfeeding. Studies in animals have not revealed harm to the fetus. There are no studies in pregnant women. Because safety in animal studies cannot assure safety in humans, this drug should not be used during pregnancy unless it is absolutely necessary. It is not known if Enbrel is excreted in human milk. Because of the potential for serious harm to the infant, a decision will be required for the mother to discontinue nursing or to remain off Enbrel.

Geriatric use. Enbrel has been successfully used to treat people over 65 years. Because older adults, in general, are at higher risk for infection, watching closely for this side effect is particularly important. (For most RA drugs, the safety and effectiveness in geriatric patients specifically has not been studied.)

Infliximab (Remicade)

Generic available: no
Usual dose: varies based on weight; intravenous infusions at weeks 0, 2, and 6, then every six to eight weeks
Effective within: two weeks to three months

Infliximab became available to treat RA in November 1999. This medication has offered a potent and exciting treatment option to patients with RA.

Like Enbrel, Remicade is a biologic TNF blocker focused on reducing the quantities of TNF in the body. Remicade reduces the amount of TNF in a slightly different way than Enbrel does. Remicade is a biogenetically engineered **antibody** that was specifically designed to attach to the TNF molecule and *permanently* inactivate it. Remicade was developed using monoclonal antibody technology (see Figure 21).

Remicade is administered intravenously by a health care professional in a two-hour outpatient infusion. There are three initial doses, and then treatments are usually given every eight weeks. In people with very active arthritis, the interval between doses can be decreased to six weeks. Some physicians give Remicade in their office. Others prefer to treat you at an infusion center or hospital. During the infusion you will be monitored by an infusion nurse. This is often a good time to read a book, listen to music, or get some well deserved relaxation.

Medical studies have shown that when used with methotrexate, Remicade effectively decreases the signs and symptoms of RA. It has also been proven to inhibit the progression of joint damage in patients with moderate or severe active RA who have had an inadequate response to methotrexate alone. At this point, Remicade is used only in combination with methotrexate.

Because Remicade is given by IV, it is treated differently than other prescriptions by most insurance plans. It is often considered a "major medical" benefit rather than part of the prescription plan. Therefore, it is a covered expense for Medicare, Medicaid, and many commercial insurance carriers. Managed care plans, or HMOs, may require a prior authorization, precertification, or a letter of medical necessity from your prescribing physician for the use of Remicade. If Remicade is being considered, call your insurance company to inquire about its specific requirements.

Side effects of Remicade. Remicade is generally well tolerated (Table 20). Because it is given intravenously, Remicade can sometimes be associated with "infusion reactions." Most reactions are mild, such as itching and stinging at the site where the IV enters the skin. Much less commonly,

Table 20
Side Effects of Remicade

Side Effects	Incidence	Side Effect Therapy
Nuisance		
Mild infusion reactions	Approx. 15%	Pretreatment with Tylenol or Benadryl
Nausea	14%	Treat nausea
Abdominal pain	8%	Seek physician's advice
Vomiting	5%	Treat symptoms; seek physician's advice
Headache	20%	Treat headache
Fatigue	6%	No specific treatment
Rash	9%	Seek physician's advice
Pain	6%	Treat pain
Itching	5%	Pretreatment with Tylenol or Benadryl
Serious		
Infusion reactions requiring discontinuation	<2%	Discontinue medication
Infections	26%	Treat infection; seek physician's advice
Lupus-like syndrome	Rare	Discontinue medication

these reactions can include rash, fever, achiness, chills, hives, chest pain, difficulty breathing, or low blood pressure. If reactions are severe, the medication must be discontinued. Many physicians "pretreat" the patient with diphenhydramine (Benadryl) and acetaminophen (Tylenol), which in many cases reduces these reactions to a tolerable level. If you are treated with Benadryl, which is sedating, you will need to discuss with your physician whether or not you should drive. In medical studies, less than 2 percent of people needed to discontinue Remicade due to infusion reactions.

Like Enbrel, Remicade can affect your immune system, which can increase the risk of infections in some people with RA. The manufacturer cautions that "there are reports of serious infections, including sepsis and tuberculosis that may be life-threatening. So, if you are prone to or have a history of infections, currently have one, or develop one while taking Remicade, tell your doctor right away. Also tell your doctor before beginning treatment if you have had close contact with, or if you have had past exposure to, people with tuberculosis, or if you have any other reason to believe you may be at risk" (Remicade package insert [2000]). Before starting Remicade, your physician may recommend a TB skin test to check for latent, or "hidden," tuberculosis. Latent tuberculosis should be treated before starting Remicade. A chest x-ray may also be requested to look for signs of past TB. There have also been reports of unusual fungal infections and other opportunistic infections in people receiving Remicade.

Treatment with Remicade may result in the development of *autoantibodies*, antibodies that are directed against one's own body. Usually, these autoantibodies cause no harm. Rarely, though, people with autoantibodies develop a lupus-like syndrome, and treatment should be discontinued.

Before starting Remicade therapy, discuss the following with your physician:

· Any poorly controlled diabetes, open wounds, signs of infection, predisposition to infection, or history of serious infections
· Any risk of tuberculosis now or in the past; a TB skin test is recommended

While receiving Remicade:

· During the infusion, make the nurse aware of any symptoms you experience, but in particular chills, chest tightness, shortness of breath, flushing, hives, itching, or dizziness.
· Contact your physician immediately with fever, chills, cough, or other symptoms of infection.
· If you develop increased achiness, pain with breathing, mouth sores, sensitivity to the sun, or a rash, contact your doctor.

· Do *not* get any "live" vaccines. Flu shots are a form of "killed" or inactivated vaccine and *should* be given in most circumstances. Pneumonia vaccinations are generally recommended.

Pregnancy and breastfeeding. Because of its specificity to humans, Remicade cannot be studied in pregnant animals. It is not known if it can cause harm to the fetus. Remicade should only be given to pregnant women if it is clearly needed. It is not known whether Remicade is excreted in breast milk. Because other antibodies can be found in breast milk, and because of the potential for harm to nursing infants, a decision should be made to stop the medication or to stop nursing.

Geriatric use. In medical studies, there was no difference in safety between younger and older adults' responses to Remicade. Because older adults are at higher risk for infection, watching closely for this side effect is particularly important.

Adalimumab (Humira)

Generic available: no
Usual dose: self-administered injections every two weeks
Effective within: two to twelve weeks

Until very recently, adalimumab, previously known as D2E7, was in Phase III trials (final phase of a clinical study—see Chapter 21). We now know that it will be released in 2003 as Humira. Like Remicade, Humira is a *monoclonal antibody* against TNF (see Figure 21). Unlike Remicade, which is made partly with mouse proteins, Humira is a fully human protein, and this is expected to lessen its side effects. Also it is given by self-administered injection and not by intravenous infusion.

In medical studies, Humira has been shown to be highly effective as a monotherapy or as a part of combination therapy with other DMARDs. Early reports reveal significant improvement in pain, swelling, and stiffness. This new TNF blocker is an exciting addition to our biologic armamentarium. The effectiveness of Humira is expected to be very similar to Enbrel and Remicade, which have been tremendously helpful in controlling RA.

Because Humira is a protein, it has to be injected by needle through the skin. The injection is given just beneath the skin (subcutaneously). Injections are required only every two weeks, which is very convenient. The area of injection is rotated from site to site (thigh, abdomen, and arm) so that no area gets too tender. Listen closely to your nurse or physician, who will teach you how to safely self-inject. It is best to have another person learn to give the injections also. Then, if your hands are too sore this care partner can help you. The helper can also inject in areas that you cannot reach. Of course, your physician and his or her staff will always be there if problems with self-administration develop.

Humira must be refrigerated at 36° to 46°F. *Do not freeze.* If you are traveling, an insulated bag or cooler will be required to keep Humira at the correct temperature. Needles and syringes must be disposed of in a puncture-resistant container. Ask your physician about disposal requirements in your community.

Because of the expense of Humira, your insurance company may require a "prior authorization," "precertification," or a "letter of medical necessity" from your prescribing physician. Call your insurance company to inquire about their specific requirements if Humira is being considered.

Side effects of Humira. The side effects of this treatment are expected to be similar to those of Enbrel and Remicade. Because it is given by subcutaneous injection, minor site reactions may occur. As with all TNF-blockers, the immune system may be affected in some individuals, leaving them at higher risk for infection. Therefore, particular attention to signs of infection is important. Always ask your physician for full instructions on what to do in the event of infection or side effects.

Before starting Humira therapy, discuss the following with your physician:

· Poorly controlled diabetes, any open wounds, signs of infection, predisposition to infection, or history of tuberculosis or other serious infections
· The need for a TB skin test and/or a chest x-ray to see if there is evidence of previous tuberculosis

While receiving Humira:

· Contact your physician if you think that you are developing any kind of infection. Humira will be temporarily discontinued in most such situations.
· If you experience severe redness, itching, pain, swelling, or any concerning symptoms at an injection site, notify your doctor.
· Never inject into a tender, red, or hard area on the skin.
· Never inject Humira that has not been properly refrigerated.
· Do not get any "live" vaccines. Flu shots are a form of "killed" or inactivated vaccine and *should* be given in most circumstances. Pneumonia vaccinations are generally recommended.
· Contact your prescribing doctor if you are planning a surgery; many physicians choose to discontinue Humira temporarily around the time of the operation, to reduce the risk of infection.

For the most current information about this new drug, check the Web site provided at the end of this chapter.

Biologic Response Modifiers against IL-1

Anakinra (Kineret)

Generic available: no
Usual dose: 100 mg, by injection once daily
Effective within: four to thirteen weeks

In November 2001 Kineret became the third biologic response modifier to be released for use in RA. It is approved by the FDA for patients with moderate to severe active RA who have failed to respond to at least one DMARD. Unlike its predecessors, which block the cytokine TNF, Kineret interferes with the cytokine interleukin-1 (IL-1), both of which stimulate inflammation. IL-1 has also been shown to be a dominant cytokine associated with the destructive changes found in RA. Kineret is a receptor antagonist, blocking receptors so that IL-1 cannot deliver its inflammation message (see Figure 19). This man-made protein is similar to the naturally occurring protein called interleukin-1 receptor antagonist (IL-1Ra).

Early studies reveal that Kineret decreases the signs and symptoms of RA, including pain and swelling. There is evidence that this medication may prove to be very valuable in preventing injury to the cartilage and bones that surround joints affected by RA. Kineret can be used alone or in combination with methotrexate or other DMARDs. At the time of this writing, it is advised that Kineret not be used with biologics that block TNF (such as Enbrel and Remicade). This is due to concern that if both IL-1 and TNF are blocked at the same time, risk of infection will be dangerously increased by so much interference with natural immune system responses. Formal studies looking at this type of combination are under way. There is hope that a combination of cytokine blockers will have tremendous effectiveness in treating RA. Full understanding of potential side effects is needed before recommending biologic combination therapy, however.

Kineret is given by subcutaneous injections (injections just below the skin). It is given as a daily injection. Each dose comes in a prefilled syringe; no mixing is necessary. Your nurse or health professional will teach you how to safely give yourself an injection. Kineret can also be administered using a SimpleJect Auto-Injector System, which makes self-injection easy and more comfortable.

Like other biologics, Kineret is a protein and must be stored in the refrigerator at 36° to 46°F. Do not let it freeze. Do not use a dose that has been at room temperature for longer than 24 hours. If you are traveling,

Table 21
Side Effects of Kineret

Side Effects	Incidence	Side Effect Therapy
Nuisance		
Injection site reaction	71%	See text
Headache	12%	Treat headache
Nausea	8%	Treat nausea
Diarrhea	7%	Treat diarrhea
Abdominal pain	5%	Treat symptoms
Flu-like symptoms	6%	Treat symptoms
Sinusitis	7%	Treat symptoms
Serious		
Infection (most mild)	40%	Discontinue medication; treat infection
Serious infections	2%	Discontinue medication; treat infection

an insulated bag or cooler will be required to keep Kineret at the correct temperature. For safety, emptied syringes must be discarded in a puncture-resistant container. Ask your doctor or nurse how to dispose of the container in your community.

Because Kineret treatment is expensive, your insurance company may require a prior authorization, precertification, or a letter of medical necessity from your prescribing physician. If Kineret is being considered, call your insurance company to inquire about their specific requirements.

Side effects of Kineret. The most frequently reported side effect of Kineret appears to be injection-site reactions (Table 21). Most involve minor redness, bruising, swelling, or pain where the needle penetrates the skin. These reactions typically last for 14 to 28 days. Injection site reactions were described in 71 percent of patients in the early studies. Injection site swelling can be decreased by applying a cold pack on the site immediately after injection. Discuss injection site itching with your doctor, since this could be an early sign of an allergic reaction. If shots are painful, try different injection locations, such as the stomach. Make certain that the alcohol with which you prepare the injection site has dried first, to prevent stinging. Usually with some adjustment in technique, injections are well tolerated. In sensitive people, placing a cold pack on the skin *before* injections is very helpful.

As with other biologics, the side effect that causes greatest concern is the risk of infection. In studies Kineret has been associated with an increased incidence of serious infections. Your doctor should discontinue treatment with Kineret if you develop a serious infection and should not start it if you have an active infection. The safety and effectiveness of Kineret in persons whose immune systems are already suppressed and in patients with chronic infections have not been evaluated. Decreases in white blood cell counts have been seen in 8 percent of patients on Kineret. Seriously low white blood cell count (*neutropenia*) was seen in only 0.3 percent of people receiving monotherapy with Kineret. Because of this potential side effect, complete blood counts (CBCs) should be performed as a baseline and monthly for three months, then quarterly for the first year.

Before starting Kineret therapy, discuss the following with your physician:

· History of poorly controlled diabetes, open wounds, signs of infection, predisposition to infection, history of tuberculosis or other serious infections
· History of low white blood cell count
· History of hypersensitivity to *E. coli*–derived proteins
· Latex allergy, since the needle cover contains latex

While receiving Kineret:

· Contact your physician if you think that you are developing any kind of infection. Kineret will be temporarily discontinued in most situations.
· If you experience severe redness, itching, pain, swelling, or any concerning symptoms at an injection site, notify your doctor.
· Never inject into a tender, red, or hard area on the skin.
· Never inject Kineret that has not been properly refrigerated.
· Do *not* get any "live" vaccines. Flu shots are a form of "killed" or inactivated vaccine and *should* be given in most circumstances. Pneumonia vaccinations are generally recommended.

Pregnancy and breastfeeding. Reproductive studies performed on animals have not revealed problems. There are, however, no adequate studies in pregnant women. Because animal reproduction studies are not always predictive of human response, Kineret should be avoided during pregnancy. It is not known whether Kineret is secreted in breast milk. Because many drugs are secreted in human milk, caution should be exercised if Kineret is administered to nursing mothers.

Geriatric use. A total of 653 patients over the age of 65 have been treated and studied at the time of this writing. There have been no reported differences in safety or effectiveness among different age groups, but an increased sensitivity in geriatric patients cannot be ruled out. Because there is an increased risk of infections in the elderly, caution must be exercised when taking this drug.

A Biologic Medical Device for Protein A Immunoadsorption

Protein A immunoadsorption is accomplished with the Prosorba column. The Prosorba column is a therapeutic device for treating people with severe, longstanding rheumatoid arthritis whose disease has not responded to medications. It is designed to remove from the blood antibodies that are believed to be harmful for people with RA. Although this procedure was only approved for RA in March 1999, a similar procedure has been used for people with a blood condition called ITP since 1987.

This medical device consists of a plastic cylinder that contains a "filter." The procedure, called *apheresis,* is much like dialysis. During treatment, the patient will be seated or lying down while a nurse places a needle into a vein in each arm. The blood drawn from one arm passes through a machine that separates the blood cells from the plasma (the liquid portion of the blood). The plasma is then filtered through a column coated with a sandlike substance, protein A, which attracts harmful antibodies. The purified plasma is recombined with the blood cells and returned to the patient through the other arm. The procedure takes two to three hours and is performed weekly for twelve weeks. It is usually performed in a blood bank, like the Red Cross, or a hospital's apheresis center.

This procedure is reserved for only the most severe cases of RA. Approximately half of those treated have a beneficial response. That response lasts 20 to 84 weeks, with an average effectiveness of 37 weeks.

Side Effects of Prosorba Column Therapy

The most common side effects are flu-like symptoms of chills, fever, nausea, and achiness. Other potential side effects include anemia, low blood pressure, and fatigue. The Prosorba column treatment is not recommended if you are taking a form of blood pressure pill called an ACE inhibitor or if you have heart problems, high blood pressure, or blood clotting problems. Use in pregnant women has not been studied.

Medicare covers Prosorba column therapy in people who meet certain criteria. If you are considering Prosorba column therapy, contact your insurance company to find out whether this treatment is covered or special authorization procedures are required.

For More Information

The makers of Enbrel offer a toll-free patient support telephone line, an educational program called Enliven, and a Web site: 1-888-4ENBREL (1-888-436-2735); www.enbrel.com. They also provide a free educational program for people with RA called RA Access. Call 1-800-395-2270 or go to www.ra-access.com.

The makers of Kineret offer a toll-free customer support telephone line, educational programs, and a Web site: 1-866-KINERET (1-866-546-3738); www.kineretrx.com.

The makers of Remicade offer a toll-free information line, and their Web site includes a support program: 1-866-REMICARE (1-866-736-4273); www.remicade.com. On a different Web site they provide information about rheumatoid arthritis: www.rahelp.com.

The makers of Humira have created a Web site giving information about the drug: www.HUMIRA.com. On a different Web site they provide news about discoveries concerning and treatments for RA: www.RA.com.

CHAPTER 15

Corticosteroids

•

Corticosteroid medications, better known as *cortisone* or *steroids,* are useful in treating rheumatoid arthritis (RA) and a variety of other conditions, such as asthma and allergies.

Corticosteroid medications are artificially manufactured to resemble the body's own natural hormones in chemical makeup. Cortisone and hydrocortisone, two such hormones, are produced naturally by the adrenal gland. These hormones have a protective function: when a person suffers any kind of stress, the levels of these hormones increase to help the person cope physically with the particular situation.

When medications resembling the body's natural cortisone are taken in larger amounts than the body normally produces, inflammation is markedly decreased. For this reason, corticosteroid medications can be an important part of the treatment of RA.

Oral Corticosteroids

Corticosteroids were first prescribed for patients with RA in the 1940s, when Dr. Phillip Hench introduced cortisone to the world. It was immediately hailed as a "miracle drug" and the "cure" for RA. High-dose cortisone was so potent and dramatically effective in the treatment of RA that Hench and his colleague Edward Kendall received the Nobel Prize in 1950 for their work.

It soon became apparent, however, that this powerful medication caused some serious side effects, particularly at the very high doses being prescribed at that time. Because of this, most physicians in the 1960s and 1970s tried to avoid prescribing any corticosteroids. They are now being given again to treat RA (see Table 22), but physicians have become more cautious in prescribing the medication. Doctors generally heed the following guidelines when prescribing corticosteroids. The drugs are to be used

Table 22
Corticosteroids Available in Pill Form

Drug	Brand Name
Betamethasone	Celestone
Cortisone	Cortone
Dexamethasone	Decadron, Hexadrol
Methylprednisolone	Medrol
Prednisolone	(none)
Prednisone	Deltasone, Orasone
Triamcinolone	Aristocort

Note: All of the above drugs are available in generic form.

· by people whose arthritis cannot be controlled adequately by non-steroidal anti-inflammatory drugs (NSAIDs) and disease-modifying anti-rheumatic drugs (DMARDs) or by people who cannot take NSAIDs or DMARDs because of unacceptable side effects;
· in the smallest dose possible which allows the person to function (the medication should be taken in the morning as a single dose); and
· for the shortest course of treatment that is expected to be effective.

If the dose and duration of corticosteroid use can be limited, the number of side effects can be diminished significantly. Treatment of some of the rare and severe complications of RA (see Chapter 4) does involve taking larger doses of corticosteroids.

It is common practice for doctors to prescribe low-dose corticosteroids on a temporary basis. If NSAIDs prove ineffective (or cause intolerable side effects), corticosteroids can be substituted temporarily to control inflammation rapidly while awaiting the effects of the slower-acting DMARDs. This is called *bridge therapy*. After the inflammation is controlled, corticosteroids need to be tapered off slowly under a physician's guidance. One should *never* abruptly discontinue corticosteroids without the supervision of a doctor.

A further note of caution is in order here: do not let the relief provided by corticosteroids lull you into a false sense of security which causes you to think about trying to avoid treatment with DMARDs. Corticosteroids are extremely potent anti-inflammatory drugs, but they may not halt the disease process.

Side Effects of Oral Corticosteroids

The side effects of oral corticosteroids tend to be of two types: those that are immediate and those that occur as a consequence of long-term use. The frequency of these side effects varies in accordance with dose, length of treatment, and the individual. In general, small daily doses (5 mg of prednisone, for example) cause few side effects, whereas larger doses (more than 20 mg of prednisone daily) are commonly associated with side effects if continued for more than a month. Corticosteroids injected into the joints rarely cause any of the side effects listed in Table 23.

Nausea, bloating, and changes in mood are the most common immediate side effects of oral corticosteroid therapy. Long-term use can affect the muscles, bones, eyes, and hormones as well as make the person susceptible to infection. Many of the side effects resulting from long-term use will subside after corticosteroid treatment is discontinued. If a person develops a serious infection, the infection needs to be treated and the person gradually taken off the corticosteroids if possible.

Cautionary Notes

Before starting oral corticosteroid therapy discuss the following with your physician:

- A history of diabetes, glaucoma, high blood pressure, heart disease, osteoporosis, thyroid problems, stomach ulcer, or tuberculosis or positive tuberculin skin test.

While taking this medication:

- Contact your physician if you notice fever or chills; cough; sore throat; blurred vision; increased frequency, duration, or severity of headaches; eye pain; increased thirst; frequent urination; increased weakness.
- Take with meals, preferably breakfast.
- Avoid alcohol and tobacco products.
- *Never stop corticosteroids abruptly.* This can be hazardous if you have been on corticosteroids for an extended period. If you run out of medication, call your doctor immediately. Corticosteroid use must be supervised by a doctor, and discontinuation of it must also be supervised by a doctor.
- If you have a surgical or another medical procedure planned, inform

Table 23
Side Effects of Oral Corticosteroids

Side Effects	Side Effect Therapy
Immediate	
Changes in mood	
Nervousness	Reduce dosage
Insomnia	Take pill in early morning
Depression	Reduce dosage
Euphoria	No treatment necessary
Nausea	Take with meals or antacid
Changes in appearance	
Weight gain due to increased appetite	Limit fats, sweets, and baked goods; eat more fresh fruits and vegetables
Puffiness	Limit salt intake
Acne	Apply topical antibiotics
Facial hair growth	Electrolysis
Increased bruising	No treatment
Salt and fluid retention	
High blood pressure	Limit salt intake
Ankle swelling	Limit salt intake and elevate legs as often as possible
Long-term	
Osteoporosis (bone thinning)	Exercise; several possible medications: calcium, vitamin D, estrogen, calcitonin, alendronate, risedronate, raloxifene
Muscle weakness	Slowly stop medication or decrease dosage; exercise
Eye problems	
Cataracts or increased eye pressure	Close observation and treatment by an ophthalmologist
Hormonal problems	
Onset of or worsening of diabetes	Reduce dosage, consult a dietitian, take diabetes medication
Menstrual irregularities	Will return to normal after discontinuation of medication
Further changes in appearance "Moon face," "buffalo hump," stretch marks, easy bruising, fragile skin	Reduce dosage
Decreased blood supply to bones (osteonecrosis), particularly hip and knee	Evaluation by orthopedic surgeon; crutches (temporary)
Susceptibility to infections	Treat infections and slowly reduce medication after infection improves

your doctor that you are on corticosteroids. Your doctor may want to increase your dose temporarily. This is called *stress dosing*.

· If you have been on corticosteroids for more than one month, wear a medical identification tag that states that you have RA and lists the medications you are taking. This will provide valuable medical information if you are ever in an accident or become so ill that you are unable to speak for yourself.

· If you have severe nausea, vomiting, or diarrhea, you may not be absorbing your medication and should alert your physician immediately.

· If you are on long-term corticosteroids, get **bone density testing** to rule out osteoporosis, and consider treatment to prevent bone loss (see next chapter).

Pregnancy and breastfeeding. Corticosteroid use is considered *relatively* safe during pregnancy.

Corticosteroid Injections

In RA it is common for one joint to become more swollen than others or to lag behind the others in improvement. An injection of corticosteroids directly into the joint will decrease the pain, warmth, and swelling in the joint that is giving the person the most trouble. The beneficial effects generally last four to six weeks.

This is a frequently performed and effective procedure that is generally safe and well tolerated. Before the injection is administered, the skin is generally numbed with a local anesthetic. (Be certain to warn your doctor if you have ever had a reaction to local anesthetics such as Novocain or Xylocaine.) A needle is then introduced through the skin and into the joint, into which the corticosteroid is injected.

The side effects of the small amount of corticosteroid injected into the joint are minimal. If a given joint is injected no more frequently than every four months, adverse effects from the corticosteroid itself are unlikely.

Corticosteroid injection into the same joint more frequently than every four months, however, may cause joint damage. In fewer than 5 percent of patients the injected corticosteroid can actually *increase* inflammation for a short period. This is known as a *postinjection flare*. Although uncomfortable, the inflammation will decrease within two to three days. It is impossible to tell in advance of the injection whether a particular individual will suffer this side effect.

Occasionally, a dimple in the skin or a mild change in skin color will be noticed at the site of injection. These skin changes will almost always disappear with time.

As with any procedure, complications related to the procedure itself can arise. Care must be taken to avoid injuring surrounding tendons or other structures. Sterile technique is required to prevent the possibility of introducing bacteria and infection into the joint. Experienced physicians, generally **rheumatologists** or **orthopedic surgeons,** take exceptional care to avoid these complications.

What to Do After a Joint Injection

Apply ice packs to the joint for twenty minutes as soon as possible after the procedure. Rest the joint for at least forty-eight hours after the injection. Wear a **splint** if a wrist has been injected, or consider using crutches to avoid putting weight on a knee or ankle that has been injected. Avoid carrying heavy objects when a shoulder or elbow has been treated by injection.

For the first week or two after injection, avoid any activity that might stress the joint.

Call your physician if there is increased pain, swelling, or fever after forty-eight hours (increased discomfort and even swelling within the first twelve hours after an injection is common). Repeated applications of ice may help alleviate the discomfort.

CHAPTER 16

Osteoporosis Treatments

•

Many people with RA also have osteoporosis. This is related to several factors. First, RA and osteoporosis are both more common in women than in men. Second, inflammation can increase the risk of osteoporosis. Lastly, medications, particularly corticosteroids, can increase bone loss and greatly increase the risk of osteoporosis. Osteoporosis can be diagnosed easily by **bone density testing.**

Dietary and Life-Style Treatments

Eating a diet rich in calcium and vitamin D can help slow osteoporosis. Calcium is a critical building block of bone, and vitamin D helps your body absorb calcium. Calcium-rich foods include dairy products, leafy green vegetables, and shellfish. Vitamin D comes from sunlight but can also be found in fortified dairy products. Table 24 reviews the daily amounts of calcium recommended for various age groups, as formulated by the National Osteoporosis Foundation. People on corticosteroids, in addition to obtaining generous amounts of calcium in their diet, should also take 1500 mg per day of calcium in divided doses. Generally, people taking corticosteroids are advised to take low-dose vitamin D supplements. If you are on prednisone or other corticosteroids, ask your rheumatologist about vitamin D supplements.

Diet and exercise both play a role in keeping or improving bone strength. The best exercises to stimulate bone formation are weight-bearing exercises. These include brisk walking, running, jogging, weight lifting, and team sports. Weight-bearing exercise should be done three to five times per week. Rheumatoid arthritis can limit exercise options. Remember the lessons of joint protection reviewed in Chapter 8. Your physician can help you develop an exercise program that is right for you.

Table 24
National Osteoporosis Foundation Recommended
Daily Intakes of Calcium

Group	Amount (mg/day)
Children and young men (2–24 years)	1200
Men older than 24 years	1000
Women younger than 19	1600
Women 19–24 years	1200
Women 24 years to menopause	1000
Women pregnant or nursing	1600
Women after menopause	1500
Women on estrogen therapy	1000
Women not on estrogen but with risk of osteoporosis	1500

Medicinal Treatments

Hormone Replacement Therapy (HRT)

Hormone replacement therapy (HRT) is drug therapy using various forms of estrogen with or without progesterone. HRT, and the controversy over its benefits and risks, is the subject of many professional and popular books. Here we will speak only to its beneficial effects on the prevention and treatment of osteoporosis. HRT has been shown to prevent bone loss after the menopause. Many studies have also suggested that HRT likely reduces the risk of hip and spine fracture in people who already have osteoporosis. You must be cautious about taking estrogen if you have a history of phlebitis or blood clots, or if you have a strong family history of breast cancer.

Selective Estrogen Receptor Modulators (SERMs)

SERMs are estrogen-like medications that are used to prevent and treat osteoporosis in women who are past the menopause. Raloxifene (Evista) was the first medication of this type to be available in the United States. Raloxifene has been shown to reduce spine fractures but not hip fractures (at the time of this writing). Unlike hormone replacement treatment,

raloxifene does not stimulate the breast or uterus. In clinical trials, raloxifene did not increase risk of breast cancer. An infrequent side effect is
blood clots in the veins, particularly in people who are immobile for long
periods.

Bisphosphonates

Bisphosphonates are a class of medications used to prevent and treat
osteoporosis, including steroid-induced bone loss. As a group they are
among the most potent medications to treat osteoporosis. These medications are very poorly absorbed, however, and therefore must be taken first
thing in the morning on an empty stomach with a large glass of water. After taking a bisphosphonate, the person must stand or sit upright for the
next 30 minutes *before* eating breakfast.

The two bisphosphonates approved for use in the United States are al-
endronate (Fosamax) and risedronate (Actonel). Fosamax or Actonel can
be prescribed in dosages taken either daily or once a week. Both have been
proven to increase bone density as well as reduce the risk of spine and hip
fractures.

Calcitonin

Calcitonin is a man-made hormone that is also found in nature. This
hormone is not in the estrogen family. Calcitonin helps to regulate normal calcium levels and reduces bone loss. Miacalcin is a brand of salmon
calcitonin that is taken by nasal spray. It has been shown to reduce the
risk of spine fractures but not hip fractures.

Parathyroid Hormone (PTH)

Parathyroid hormone (PTH) is another nonestrogen hormone that is
found in nature. PTH has to be taken by injection, because, like the other
"biologics," it is a protein and gets digested by stomach enzymes if taken
orally. One brand of PTH is called Forteo; others are in development. This
medication is reserved for those with the most severe cases of osteoporosis.

For More Information

National Osteoporosis Foundation, 1232 22nd Street, N.W., Washington, D.C. 20037-1292; 202-223-0344; www.nof.org

The Osteoporosis Book: A Guide for Patients and Their Families, by Nancy Lane, M.D. (New York: Oxford University Press, 1999).

NIH Osteoporosis and Related Bone Diseases National Resource Center, 1232 22nd Street, N.W., Washington, D.C. 20037-1292; 202-223-0344 or toll-free 1-800-624-BONE; www.osteo.org

Beyond Medications: Other Treatments

•

Alternative and Complementary Therapies

•

As exciting as new technological and biological advances are, many people see them as only part of their treatment options. There is an ever-growing interest in nonconventional medical treatments. Historically, the medical profession has viewed with considerable skepticism treatments that have not been subjected to scientific testing. Non-Western therapies were denounced by many scientists as quackery. Despite this skepticism, people have sought *alternative treatments* when traditional medicine offered incomplete relief for chronic conditions such as rheumatoid arthritis (RA). In time, many people began to view these therapies as *complementary* to conventional medical care rather than as a replacement (or alternative) for proven treatments.

Because patients have increasingly turned to complementary therapies, physicians have had to recognize the implications of patients' using both conventional and complementary treatment options. In an effort to be helpful, many medical professionals have attempted to give informed advice to their patients, even in the absence of sound scientific research on most nonconventional treatments. Many hospitals and medical centers have acknowledged the lack of evidence in this area and have developed exploratory programs focused on *integrative medicine*. This new area of medicine is attractive to individuals who want to thoughtfully combine mainstream medicine with complementary therapies. The National Institutes of Health developed the Center for Addiction and Alternative Medicine Research to support rigorous scientific evaluation of complementary and alternative medicine. This NIH program focuses on determining the safety and effectiveness of nonconventional therapeutic approaches.

At this time, most complementary treatments are *still* unproven; hence, you are literally trying them at your own risk. Prospective treatments can range from unproven but potentially useful therapies to potentially harmful therapies. Treatments may be relatively inexpensive or very expensive. Even if a treatment is inexpensive and carries no risk of physical harm, there is the hidden cost of wasting time on unproven remedies: the person may miss the opportunity to receive proven and effective treatment during the valuable window of opportunity that occurs early in the course of RA. It is during this window of opportunity that conventional treatments are most effective in preventing structural damage from RA. Another concern is that there is very little quality control in the "dietary supplement" industry, and this creates the potential for many problems. Our advice is: *Always discuss with your doctor all therapies that you are contemplating, so that he or she can steer you away from those treatments with potential health risks.*

If complementary medicine is of interest to you, you will need to become engaged in gathering information and exploring your choices. Your physician may be willing to give you some guidance in choosing practitioners of a given treatment type, *if* he or she has had good experiences with complementary therapists. Always be honest with your doctor about treatments that you are considering. The best way to reduce your risk with unproven treatments or remedies is to *give your doctor the full story,* so he or she can follow you thoughtfully, with complete information. We, the authors, cannot endorse or recommend any complementary therapies, but we will give you some guidelines to consider when making these decisions. You will also note that many treatments just make sense and are already well on their way into mainstream medicine.

This chapter will focus on some common therapies and disciplines. It is by no means an exhaustive list or assessment. Many of the approaches discussed below involve the use of dietary supplements; these will be discussed more fully in the next chapter. Since this is such an expansive area of interest, we will only be able to scratch the surface of treatment options. Please see the resource section for this chapter for information about references dedicated to alternative and complementary treatments for arthritis.

Aromatherapy

We all know how certain aromas can help us to recall pleasant memories. Clearly, different scents can elicit different feelings and emotions. The fragrance industry has understood for decades how scent enhances attitude—"invigorating" morning shower soaps, sensual perfumes, relaxing bath salts, "power" cologne.

Aromatherapy most often uses essential oils (fragrant, highly volatile liquids produced by aromatic plants) that can be absorbed through the skin by way of massage, baths, compresses, facials, lotions, or ointments. Topical applications of several botanical oils are approved by the German government for relieving symptoms of RA. These include camphor, eucalyptus, fir needle, pine needle, and rosemary. Another approach to aromatherapy uses a vaporizer, diffuser, or steam inhaler, so the person can inhale the aroma. A therapist can present you with different scents to determine which make you feel best. Also, there are many boutiques and spas where you can test essential oils on your own. Whether it is the relaxing scent of lavender or the familiar scent of vanilla that soothes you, you can have fun experimenting. Some essential oils commonly suggested for arthritis are rosemary, lavender, juniper, eucalyptus, cypress, and ginger. Remember that relaxing the mind and body helps to alleviate discomfort. Combining your favorite scent with a warm, soothing bath and calming music can help erase even the worst day.

Do not take any of these oils internally. Essential oils should be diluted in another oil before being applied to the skin. People with eczema or sensitive skin should test a small area first to see if the oils are irritating to them. Keep the oils away from your eyes. People with asthma should discuss inhalation methods with their physician before trying them.

Ayurveda

Ayurveda has been a traditional medical system in India for more than 3,000 years. It is a comprehensive system that is still widely practiced in India. Its focus is on mental, spiritual, and physical balance. It approaches illness through life-style modifications and a wide range of natural therapies. According to Ayurveda, people, like the universe, are made of five elements and the soul. The five elements in their biological form in the body are known as *doshas*. All functions of the body and mind are dependent on the state of these doshas. Different doshas are associated with different physical and personality characteristics. Customized treatments are based on these body-soul-energy "types." Programs include individualized herbs and supplements, meditation, massage, exercise, and purification regimens that may involve fasting, baths, and purging. In Ayurveda, diet, meditation, and healthy life-style practices promote physical and spiritual well-being. Be very cautious about unmonitored fasting or purging methods. Some Ayurvedic herb mixtures are also an area for concern, because there is no standard of quality control (see next chapter).

Yoga is a practice that stems from ancient Ayurvedic healing. It is often used as part of an Ayurvedic program to bring "union" to the body, mind, and spirit, but it can be performed without embracing the full Ayurvedic principles and practices. There are several variations of yoga practice. They have in common elements of stretching, postures, relaxation, meditation, and breathing techniques. Studies have shown that yoga can bring improvement in flexibility, strength, equilibrium, and stamina to healthy and ill persons. Although there are not many studies reviewing yoga and RA, one small study (Haslock et al., 1994) did show improved physical strength and acceptance in the study participants.

The focus on gentle stretching and strengthening is consistent with joint protection principles. Breath awareness and relaxation techniques in general help relieve stress and control pain. Yoga is best learned from an *experienced* teacher, because improper positioning can be harmful. Let your instructor know which joints are inflamed; specific yoga postures can be modified for you or supports can be used to prop up inflamed joints. For instance, exercises can be performed while sitting in a chair rather than on the floor. Review yoga positions with your rheumatologist; individuals with significant joint damage or joint replacements may have limitations.

Bodywork

Multiple forms and styles of bodywork can be used to relieve pain and tension. Massage is the most common. Massage is defined as the manual manipulation of soft tissues of the body by movements such as rubbing, kneading, rolling, or pressing for therapeutic purposes. Manipulation of the tissues increases blood flow and warmth. Common techniques include Swedish, sport, acupressure, trigger point, myofascial release, deep tissue, and rolfing.

If you are having a severe flare, any bodywork may be too uncomfortable for you. If you are not too sore or swollen, however, and your physician agrees, massage may be an option. Most qualified massage therapists know several techniques and can adjust to your specific problems. *Always tell your therapist that you have RA* and which joints are involved. If you are not sure what type of massage to ask for, we would recommend Swedish massage, with its gentle stroking and kneading motions. This technique promotes circulation of blood and lymph and muscle relaxation without harsh motions, rigorous stretching or overzealous manipulation, which can hurt tender or vulnerable joints.

Acupressure, like acupuncture, uses acupoint locations on meridians (see "Chinese Medicine" below). Pressure on these points is incorporated into general massage. Japanese acupressure, called *shiatsu,* also focuses on acupoints. Shiatsu is usually practiced on a floor mat and can involve stretching, which may present a problem for those with significant RA.

Deep tissue techniques, myofascial release, and rolfing involve deeper massage, which helps many people but may be too aggressive for those with very tender joints and muscles. More focused forms of bodywork include reflexology and craniosacral therapy.

When you are having any sort of bodywork, *speak up right away if what you are experiencing is painful or uncomfortable in any way.*

Breathing Techniques, Breath Therapy, or Breathwork

It may seem unusual to consider breathing as a form of therapy, but breathing techniques are an important part of many complementary and alternative therapies (for example, massage, yoga, tai chi). Breathwork is closely linked to most forms of relaxation therapy. Many people believe that breathing exercises are so important that even alone they should be considered a form of therapy. During our busy lives, we mostly survive with quick, shallow breaths. Each time we yawn—an automatic, full, deep, diaphragmatic breath—our bodies are trying to tell us that we need something more. Breathing exercises are beneficial in bringing oxygen to tissues, promoting blood flow, and enhancing other physiologic functions, such as digestion.

Breath is the simplest technique that connects the body and mind. Deep breathing techniques have been shown to slow the heart rate, promote relaxation, improve emotional well-being, and enhance vitality. Focused breathing brings you clearly into the moment. Many people find that breathwork, particularly when combined with meditation, provides an opportunity for self-discovery or spiritual awakening. Sounds almost too good to be true, doesn't it?

Breathing techniques include three phases: inhalation, retention, and exhalation. Whenever you are feeling stressed, take a long, deep breath through your nose; make your diaphragm move rather than your chest as you breathe in; hold the air in a few seconds and breathe out slowly through your mouth. You will be surprised how even a few breaths make a difference. As aptly described by Andrew Weil, M.D., author and expert in breathwork: "The simplest and most powerful technique for protecting your health is absolutely free—and literally right under your nose."

Chinese Medicine

Chinese medicine involves ancient principles and practices. The flow of vital life energy, called *Qi* (pronounced chee), is central to this discipline. Qi flows in channels called *meridians* that can become blocked, causing your Qi to be out of balance. When Qi is out of balance, illness can occur. Arthritis is believed to be a deficiency of Qi. The goal of Chinese medicine is to balance the yin and yang—opposing forces of nature. Chinese treatments used to balance the flow of Qi include acupuncture, acupressure, tai chi, Qi-gong, and Chinese herbs.

Acupuncture

Acupuncture has become a very popular treatment in the United States in the past decade. Treatments are still given in traditional Chinese medicine environments but have also found their way into conventional treatment arenas such as pain clinics and physicians' offices. More than 4,000 doctors (including this book's first author) have completed a recognized acupuncture training program in the United States. Acupuncture involves inserting extremely thin solid needles at specific points (acupoints) along meridians to balance the flow of Qi and improve health, according to Chinese theory. How acupuncture works is not completely understood. Western researchers propose that acupuncture may stimulate deep sensory nerves that tell the body to release natural painkillers, called endorphins. Animal studies have shown an increase in cortisol, a natural antiinflammatory agent, after acupuncture treatment. To date, there has been no scientifically valid study that proves acupuncture can halt the effects of RA.

Almost all Western practicing acupuncturists use disposable needles, and you should not accept treatment with reused needles. Definitely make the acupuncturist aware of any artificial joints you have, so he or she can use extra care. Treatments are not as painful as you might expect. You may feel a slight pinch that lasts a few seconds. Generally speaking, it takes at least four treatments before any improvement is seen. If you are fearful of needles, you may want to consider acupressure. *Acupressure* uses similar points but instead of needles uses firm sustained pressure to "open channels." Techniques of acupressure are often incorporated into massage or bodywork.

Tai Chi

A relative newcomer, for Chinese medicine, tai chi dates back only a few hundred years. Originating as a martial arts practice, it has evolved into a relaxation technique, self-healing practice, and fitness activity. When not used for self-defense, its movements are slow, circular, rhythmic, flowing, and dancelike. It also encompasses elements of meditation and breathing techniques to promote harmony of mind and body. It can also promote flexibility, vitality, and increased power of attention. Western practitioners have shown that it can improve balance, decrease falls, promote relaxation, and decrease pain.

This form of therapy, with its controlled movements and graceful gestures, may prove very valuable to people with RA if it does not include strong martial arts elements (Kirsteins et al., 1991). In fact, a tai chi program devised for arthritis patients is offered by the Arthritis Foundation of Australia (see end of chapter). Tai chi can be taught in several styles, variations, and techniques. It is always best to learn tai chi from an experienced instructor. A qualified teacher with knowledge about rheumatoid arthritis can determine if these techniques are appropriate for you or if modifications are possible. Review all movements with your doctor and follow our exercise precautions, listed in Chapter 9.

Qi-gong

Qi-gong is a self-healing art that dates back at least 3,000 years. *Qi* (energy) and *gong* (skill) together literally mean "the skill of cultivating vital energy." Qi-gong, referred to as "the healing dance of life," combines the principles of movement, posture, breathing, relaxation, and visualization. Qi-gong involves gentle body movement and meditation with slow adjustments in body posture. Breath and movement are synchronized. Regular practice of Qi-gong can improve both balance and strength. With its slow and relaxed motions, Qi-gong is less physically challenging than tai chi and may be more suitable for people with severe RA. Visualizations are used to guide the energy, enhance the mind-body connection, promote spiritual self-development, and promote healing. There are several variations on the practice of Qi-gong. As always, find an experienced teacher who understands RA.

Chinese Herbs

Like Ayurvedic herbs, Chinese herbs are generally mixtures of various herbs and other substances. The exact amount of active ingredients in a preparation is difficult to determine, due to variations in the quality of herbs. The potential for contaminants in mixtures has also caused concern (see "Chinese Herbs" in next chapter).

Music and Sound Therapy

It probably sounds silly to consider music a form of therapy. Intuitively, we all realize that different types of music elicit different feelings and emotions. Music and sound therapy involves the controlled use of sounds in the treatment of disorders. Soothing music can promote relaxation and relieve stress. Familiar environmental sounds, like a running stream, a waterfall, or birds singing, can calm the mind and create a positive mood.

Researchers have suggested that soothing sounds can stimulate production of endorphins, the body's natural painkillers. As simple as these notions are, we infrequently take advantage of this simple remedy. So, take some time to listen to your favorite music today.

Other Mind-Body Therapies

Although often considered in the realm of complementary medicine, the importance of the mind-body connection is thousands of years old and is represented in ancient Eastern and Western medical systems and religions. Eastern practices of *yoga, tai chi,* and *Qi-gong* rely heavily on mind-body practices.

In the last few decades Western societies have incorporated these concepts into mainstream medicine. Biofeedback, for example, is commonly used to help people cope with pain, anxiety, and tension. People learn skills that help them identify and respond to changes in their own bodies. In Chapter 7 we addressed some techniques that have been used to decrease stress, anxiety, and tension. You may wish to read this chapter again, to remind yourself of the benefits of *meditation, biofeedback, imagery, progressive relaxation,* and *prayer.*

In the 1990s the interest in healing practices has soared in the West. Individuals such as Andrew Weil, Deepak Chopra, and Carolyn Myss have written on healing as a natural internal power that we all possess. The theories and practices by which we can enlist these inner resources are as variable as each individual who seeks information. There are literally thousands of books, lectures, and tapes that focus on healing. They all have in common the basic principle of developing your own inner resources to get to a stronger, better place both mentally and physically. Getting there is a journey worth taking. Whether through traditional practices of faith and prayer or through less common spiritual exercise, tapping the power of your inner self will help you master your RA, as well as other challenges that life throws your way. Again, as powerful as these strategies may be, they work best as *an adjunct to* and not *a replacement for* conventional treatment.

Naturopathy

Naturopathy is medicine based on "natural remedies." Naturopathic medicine tends to focus on healthy life-style, nutrition, and exercise. Naturopathic treatments use herbs, supplements, counseling, massage, spinal manipulation, and diverse other approaches. The naturopathic physician (N.D.) usually undergoes a four-year training program. These practitioners may also specialize in other types of therapy, such as acupuncture and homeopathy. Many people appreciate the naturopathic emphasis on symptom control, exercise, and diet. A well-informed N.D. will encourage you to continue your conventional medications and to ask your rheumatologist about any herbs, supplements, or exercise recommendations. A naturopathic doctor who leads you away from conventional assessment and treatment should be avoided, since valuable time can be lost.

Spa Therapy and Hydrotherapy

Spas are one of the oldest forms of therapy for patients with arthritis. The practice of "taking the waters," bathing in and drinking mineral waters, is ancient and widespread. The question is whether the benefit is from the hydrotherapy or from the mineral and other natural ingredients in the natural spas. Hydrotherapy involves the therapeutic use of water, steam, or ice. Techniques include baths, compresses, showers, steam rooms, and whirlpools. Hydrotherapy alone has been shown to increase strength, balance, and range of motion of joints. Again, whether there are additional benefits of natural spas is less clear. There has been speculation that everything from natural radon to Dead Sea bath salts have special "healing" properties.

Homeopathy

The theory of homeopathy was developed by a German physician, Samuel Hahneman, in the 1700s. His theory was based on three principles: the "law of similars," the "minimum dose," and "the single remedy." The theory holds that if a large amount of a substance causes specific symptoms in a healthy person, smaller amounts of the same substance can treat those same symptoms in someone who is ill. People are given minute amounts of substances that would *cause* illness if given in larger amounts. These highly diluted substances theoretically stimulate the body into a healing mode. Treatments are prescribed based on symptoms and personality rather than on the disease itself. Remedies are made from plants, minerals, and animals.

Very little research has been performed using this type of treatment for RA. There have been small, poorly designed studies with conflicting results. A recent English study (Fisher and Scott, 2001) found no evidence that homeopathy improved symptoms or signs of RA. Professionals who practice homeopathy include naturopathic physicians (N.D.s), doctors of medicine (M.D.s), dentists, chiropractors, and acupuncturists.

Guidelines for Evaluating Unproven Treatments

Educate yourself using trusted resources. When considering alternative forms of therapy, avoid:

· Treatments that offer *miracles* and *cures*. If it sounds too good to be true, it usually is.
· Treatments for which testimonials (patients' stories) are the only proof of the therapy's effectiveness
· "Secret" treatments, ones which you are urged not to discuss with other people

When choosing a practitioner:

· Personal references are always best. Start by asking your doctor, support group, or local Arthritis Foundation.
· The state or national credentialing organization for a particular discipline will sometimes provide referrals.
· Ask for credentials, certifications, or license information.
· Find out where the therapist trained.
· Find out how long the therapist has been in practice and where.
· Find out how much experience the therapist has had with RA patients.
· Do not pay in advance for a series of treatments; pay as you go.
· Make sure the therapist is willing to work with your conventional doctor.
· Speak with your regular doctor before you begin any form of treatment.

Be skeptical of practitioners who:

· Have a "conspiracy theory" for mainstream medicine and pharmaceutical companies; particularly avoid those who ask you to stop your medications
· Sell high-priced supplements, particularly if the ingredients are not listed
· Recommend computer-scored "nutrient deficiency tests" as a basis for selling you vitamins and supplements
· Offer pseudoscientific diagnostic tests that cannot be obtained from your regular doctor
· Engage in multiple-level marketing, that is, ask you to be a salesperson for them
· Have moved several times in a short span of years

For More Information

A comprehensive and balanced guide to alternative medicine, including treatments using food supplements, is *The Arthritis Foundation's Guide to Alternative Therapies,* by Judith Horstman (Atlanta, Ga.: Arthritis Foundation, 1999).

For further information on complementary and alternative medicine for practitioners and the public, contact NIH National Center for Complementary and Alternative Medicine (NCCAM), P.O. Box 8218, Silver Spring, Md. 20907-8218; toll-free 1-888-644-6226. The NCCAM Clearinghouse is an NIH-funded information service for the public, to enhance understanding of complementary and alternative medicine. Its Web site is http://nccam.nih.gov.

An excellent resource on breathwork is *Breathing: The Master Key to Self-Healing,* by Andrew Weil, M.D. (Louisville, Colo.: Sounds True, 1999). It is also available on CD and audio tape.

A video tape and handbook on tai chi endorsed by the Arthritis Foundation of Australia are titled *Tai Chi for Arthritis,* by Paul Lam, M.D. (2000). The author is an Australian doctor and tai chi teacher.

Two books describing yoga specifically designed for people with disabilities are *Gentle Yoga: For People with Arthritis, Stroke Damage, MS, or People in Wheelchairs,* by Lorna Bell and Eudora Seyfer (Berkeley, Calif.: Celestial Arts, 1987); and *Gentle Yoga: Guide to Low-Impact Exercise,* by Lorna Bell and Eudora Seyfer (Berkeley, Calif.: Celestial Arts, 1990).

The American Yoga Association has joined with the Arthritis Foundation and Aventis Pharmaceuticals to launch an on-line yoga guide for RA patients. The guide, "Remain Active with RA," includes exercises aimed at range of motion, muscle strengthening, and endurance. See the Web site, http://www.RAacademy.com.

Two books on the power of the mind-body connection and self-healing are *Simple Abundance: A Daybook of Comfort and Joy,* by Sarah Ban Breathnach (New York: Warner Books, 1995); and *Inner Peace for Busy People,* by Joan Borysenko (Carlsbad, Calif.: Hay House, 2001).

CHAPTER 18

Nutrition: Diets, Nutrients, and Food Supplements

•

Nutrition and RA

The idea that a person can completely control rheumatoid arthritis (RA) by dietary means is very compelling to most people. It certainly would be exciting if we could achieve a complete remission through diet manipulation and "natural" means. Unfortunately, at this time there is no proven diet that will definitely halt the progression of RA. However, the bookstore shelves offer many volumes promising "cures" with the right dietary change. Although most of these claims lack scientific basis, there may be beneficial dietary practices that we are only beginning to understand. Researchers have become increasingly interested in foods and their constituents and how particular foods may improve general health and specific medical conditions. First, we will review the scientifically tested fundamentals of a nutritious diet. Then, we will address dietary changes suggested or advertised to be beneficial. Finally, we will look at the most popular dietary supplements, which include vitamins and minerals, herbs, and other supplements.

Please remember that *only* the disease-modifying antirheumatic drugs (**DMARDs**) and biologic response modifiers (**BRMs**) have been *proven* to halt the progression of rheumatoid arthritis. The following information is provided to help you make sense of the tremendous amount of information you will be exposed to by commercial interests, Internet searches, and well-meaning friends. Some of the practical dietary information can be safely incorporated into your daily meal planning. Any supplementation or significant dietary change should be discussed thoroughly with your physician. Until we have more scientific information on dietary manipulation and its effects on RA, we suggest you follow a healthy, balanced diet that promotes a healthy weight.

A Well-Balanced, Nutritious Diet

A person's diet must be both well balanced and nutritious to maintain energy stores and to keep muscles functioning well enough to protect the joints. Ideally, the number of calories you consume each day will maintain your healthy body weight. In some people with very active RA, weight loss may be a problem. More commonly, however, weight gain is the problem. There are several reasons for this. Taking medications that increase appetite (for example, corticosteroids) can result in weight gain. In addition, many people with RA have muscle loss, which decreases the body's metabolic rate; it doesn't burn as many calories, so it doesn't need as many. Finally, arthritis often limits physical activity, resulting in decreased calorie use.

A nutritionally balanced diet consists of a variety of foods from different food groups. Nutrition scientists have developed the "Dietary Guidelines for Americans" and "The Food Guide Pyramid." Developed by the United States Department of Agriculture and supported by the Department of Health and Human Services, they form a research-based dietary system. The emphasis of these guidelines is on reducing fat and unhealthy foods and encouraging wise food choices. These principles also make good sense for people with RA.

The Food Guide Pyramid

Each food group in the pyramid contains nutrients that we need. But the pyramid shape is designed to encourage us to choose foods from the five food groups at the base of the pyramid. See Figure 22 for the five food groups and general recommendations on servings per day. At the tip of the pyramid is the group that contains fats, oils, and sweets—foods we enjoy but should eat sparingly. Different foods contain different nutrients. If you find that you are eliminating all or most of any one food group, you will need professional guidance to make sure that you are making up for the nutrients in other ways.

For each of the food groups the pyramid offers a range of servings that varies according to calorie requirements. The National Academy of Sciences has established some *very general* recommendations about calorie consumption:

· sedentary women and some older adults: 1,600 calories
· active women and sedentary men: 2,200 calories
· some very active men and women: 2,800 calories

See Table 25.

Most people with active RA would require between 1,600 and 2,200

Food Guide Pyramid
A Guide to Daily Food Choices

Fats, Oils, & Sweets
USE SPARINGLY

KEY
◨ Fat (naturally   ▼ Sugars
   occurring and added)   (added)

These symbols show fat and
added sugars in foods.

Milk, Yogurt,
& Cheese
Group
2-3 SERVINGS

Meat, Poultry, Fish,
Dry Beans, Eggs,
& Nuts Group
2-3 SERVINGS

Vegetable
Group
3-5 SERVINGS

Fruit
Group
2-4 SERVINGS

Bread, Cereal,
Rice, & Pasta
Group
**6-11
SERVINGS**

Source: U.S. Department of Agriculture/U.S. Department of Health and Human Services

Figure 22

calories. If you find that you are gaining weight, decrease the number of calories but maintain balance among the food groups. Lowering fat or sugar is always the fastest and safest way to calorie reduction. Low-fat diets may also ease the symptoms of RA (Lucas et al., 1981). If you are trying to lose weight, try not to go below the number of servings in the five major food groups.

Fats, Oils, and Sugars

Recommendation: use sparingly

Some fat is necessary in your diet, and it is impossible to avoid all fat, because fat is a component of foods in important nutrient groups, like dairy and meat. Fats supply nutrients called essential fatty acids and are

Table 25
Sample Daily Recommendations from the Pyramid Guide

Food Groups	Person's Caloric Need		
	1600 calories	2200 calories	2800 calories
Grain group servings	6	9	11
Vegetable group servings	3	4	5
Fruit group servings	2	3	4
Milk group servings	2–3	2–3	2–3
Meat group (ounces)	5	6	7
Total fat (grams)	53	73	93
Total added sugars (teaspoons)	6	12	18

important for absorption of fat-soluble vitamins A, D, E, and K. All fats add calories to your diet. Total fat calories should be responsible for no more than 30 percent of your calories. For example, if your diet permits, 1,950 calories per day, no more than 585 calories (30 percent) should come from fat. Each gram of fat has 9 calories. Dividing 585 calories by 9, you see that you are allowed 65 grams of fat per day.

Saturated fats are found in animal fat, dairy products, and some vegetable oils, such as coconut and palm oil. These fats are the most harmful to consume in excess, because they can increase cholesterol and the risk of heart disease. This type of fat should be limited to less than 10 percent of your total calorie intake, or one-third of your daily fat intake. Foods high in *trans fatty acids* also tend to raise cholesterol. These foods include those high in partially hydrogenated vegetable oils, like shortenings. Commercially fried foods and some bakery goods use these fats in high amounts. *Unsaturated fats* do not raise cholesterol but are still high in calories. We describe below the fats called *omega-3 fatty acids* which may have additional anti-inflammatory benefits. Choosing foods and oils with these fatty acids may be particularly advantageous for people with RA. Fat grams from omega-3 oils will still have to be counted in the dietary plan, like any other dietary fat.

Getting used to a low-fat diet requires exploring new ideas, learning more about foods, and making consistently wise choices. Check all ingredient labels for the type and grams of fat contained. Choose lean meats and skim milk. Consider low-fat toppings, such as salsa, lemon juice, and herbs. Use low-fat cooking methods. Choose sliced turkey or chicken breast over high-fat luncheon meats.

Sugars occur naturally in nutrient-rich foods such as milk, fruits, and some vegetables. Added sugar, however, is a large source of empty calories for many Americans. It is often present in the bread and cereal group and is used in the processing of syrups for canned fruits. Most foods containing added sugar increase calories and risk of dental disease with little nutritional benefit. Good examples include soft drinks, candy, and most desserts.

When planning your diet, remember that balance is the key. Favorite but "forbidden" foods may be eaten very occasionally if your doctor agrees.

Bread, Cereals, Rice, and Pasta

Recommendation: six to eleven servings daily

Carbohydrates are an excellent source of energy. They can also be an excellent source of fiber, minerals, and vitamins. Particularly important are whole-grain foods, such as certain breads and cereals. Grains vary in nutrient content, so choose a variety of grains. High-fiber carbohydrates promote proper bowel function. Soluble fiber from whole oats may reduce heart disease when eaten with a diet low in saturated fats. High-fiber foods also help you feel full. Whole-grain products are naturally low in fat and high in fiber. Many baked goods and pastries, however, use refined flour, which is low in fiber. Also, commercial baked goods are frequently high in fat and sugar. Most Americans don't consume enough fiber. The American Dietetic Association recommends 20 to 30 grams of fiber daily for most people. Use the nutrition facts label to help choose grains high in fiber and low in sugar, saturated fat, and sodium. (Remember: whole-grain noodles are healthful, but drenching them in cream sauce makes them a high-calorie, high-fat dish.)

Vegetables

Recommendation: three to five servings daily

Vegetables provide critical vitamins, such as vitamins A and C, and folate, as well as minerals, such as iron and magnesium. Vegetables, particularly when eaten raw, are also important sources of fiber. Different vegetables add different nutrients. Dark green leafy vegetables, orange vegetables (carrots, pumpkins), and tomatoes are good sources of vitamin A. Broccoli, peppers, tomatoes, cabbage, potatoes, and leafy greens are good sources of vitamin C. Folate is found in dry beans, dark leafy vegetables, and green peas. White and sweet potatoes are good sources of potassium. Vegetables with the deepest, brightest colors usually are the most nutritious. Choosing foods with different colors will give you different food pigments. Pigments contain phytochemicals, which can act as **antioxidants**. Consuming a variety of antioxidants is beneficial.

Fruits

Recommendation: two to four servings daily

Fruits are important sources of vitamins A and C and potassium. Fruits, particularly unpeeled and raw, are an important source of fiber. Orange-colored fruits (mango, cantaloupe, apricots) are high in vitamin A and other carotenoids. Citrus fruits, kiwi, strawberries, and cantaloupe are loaded with vitamin C. Blue or purple fruits are high in antioxidants called anthocyanins. Plan a diet with various colors of fruits in order to get a broad range of pigments and antioxidants. Choose fresh or frozen fruits and juices, but note that some canned and some frozen fruits are high in sugar, because they are processed in a sweetened syrup.

Meat, Poultry, Fish, Dry Beans, Eggs, and Nuts

Recommendation: two to three servings; total five to seven ounces of lean meat, poultry, or fish

This group of foods provides needed proteins, B vitamins, iron, and zinc. Trimming away all visible fat is important. Choose leaner cuts of beef, pork, and veal. Remove the skin of chicken and turkey. Broil or roast meats rather than frying them. Choose low-fat marinades. Legumes (beans), including kidney and pinto beans, are good protein sources.

Adding some meatless meals featuring beans (kidney, pinto, black beans) to your diet will bring variety as well as new nutrients into your meal planning. Be careful to avoid spreads, oils, and dressings with excessive fat.

Milk, Yogurt, and Cheese

Recommendation: two to three servings

Milk products provide protein, vitamins, and minerals, particularly calcium. Adequate calcium intake is important with RA, because of the risk of **osteoporosis**. Choose skim milk and low-fat or no-fat yogurts and cheese, including cottage cheese.

Dietary Guidelines for Americans

In summary, for most Americans, the U.S. Department of Agriculture and the Department of Health and Human Services recommend the following:

· Eat a variety of foods.
· Balance the food you eat with physical activity; maintain or improve your weight.
· Choose a diet with plenty of grain products, vegetables, and fruits.
· Choose a diet low in fat, saturated fat, and cholesterol.
· Choose a diet moderate in sugars.
· Choose a diet moderate in salt and sodium.
· If you drink alcoholic beverages, do so in moderation.

They also advise us to drink at least five eight-ounce glasses of water per day, to read food labels when we make selections of food, and to increase our intake of dietary fiber.

Special Diets

The promise of dietary "cures" for RA is alluring, and books touting such cures are prevalent. Although there is much written on this subject, scientific studies on the impact of diets are scant, often poorly designed, and inconclusive. One need not read long before finding that the supposedly curative dietary strategies conflict with each other. However, within each strategy, there may be elements that will prove helpful for *some* individuals. Researchers are looking very closely at diet and its relationship to arthritis. Patients and physicians will be eager to hear the results. There are two basic principles on which diet therapies are based.

The first principle is that *some* individuals have a sensitivity to specific foods, and that eating those foods aggravates rheumatoid arthritis. The diet strategy in these situations is to *avoid* the offending food. Suggested culprits include dairy, wheat, corn, beef, pork, and eggs. Eliminating foods that contain solanine (tomatoes, white potatoes, peppers, eggplant, and other vegetables in the "nightshade family") has helped some individuals. Food additives, such as MSG (monosodium glutamate), and food dyes have also been considered suspect. In 2001, Finnish researchers suggested a link between consuming decaffeinated beverages and developing RA (Mikuls et al., 2002). In the past, decaffeinated coffee was processed with chemical solvents, which may explain this finding. That is no longer the case.

With the growing interest in nutrition, other possible linkages will likely be questioned and reported. From what we know *at this time,* food sensitivities appear to play a role in only a *small portion* of people with RA.

The second principle, in contrast, is that by *adding* certain healthy foods to the diet, arthritis symptoms might be decreased. Supplementing the diet with specific foods that have antioxidant and anti-inflammatory effects helps lessen symptoms of RA. This is a very exciting area, and science has only scratched the surface of its potential. By initiating scientifically validated research studies, we hope to identify these healing foods and determine why they help.

Be advised against following any long-term, severe dietary restriction without the guidance of a certified nutritionist or licensed professional. Discuss any significant dietary change with your physician.

Elimination Diets

Elimination diets are based on the premise that some foods contain ingredients that cause or aggravate arthritis and that the culprit(s) can be determined by systematic elimination of suspect foods. Elimination diets can be conservative—removing one food at a time while observing symptoms—or rigorous, starting with a very limited diet (or even fasting) and slowly adding back foods one at a time. The second version clearly needs to be guided by a licensed professional. In some studies, individuals have been able through elimination diets to identify foods that aggravate their arthritis symptoms. Common offending foods include wheat (**gluten**-containing foods), corn, pork, oranges, and milk. If you are going to pursue this type of diet, it is best to work with a health professional knowledgeable about food allergies, to make sure that you are meeting your nutritional requirements while you are limiting foods. Remember, if you remove a group of foods, you need to replace its vital nutrients in other ways. For example, when removing dairy products, add calcium and vitamin D supplements. Elimination diets can be harmful, particularly when you give up nutritious foods at the time you need them most.

Fasting

In several studies, fasting has been shown to reduce the *symptoms* of RA. Unfortunately, the benefits appear to be short-lived, and symptoms return when a regular diet is resumed. A German review of this topic was published (Muller et al., 2001). Muller found four studies showing that fasting, followed by a vegetarian diet, was associated with some benefit. Since fasting is not sustainable and may be harmful, it is *not recommended* as an option and clearly should not be attempted without your doctor's permission and supervision. A more exciting angle, however, is that researchers are looking at fasting patients to determine what changes may be responsible for reducing inflammation. One Norwegian study (Fraser et al., 2000) showed that an inflammatory *cytokine,* called IL-6, was reduced in these patients. Fasting is not practical, but finding practical ways to duplicate this effect would be a great breakthrough.

Vegetarian Diets

There are several degrees of vegetarian diets. Many people choose not to follow a strict vegan diet (no dairy, eggs, fish, or meat). Some may eat dairy products (lactovegetarian), eggs (ovovegetarian), or fish (pescovegetarian). Researchers at the University of Kupio in Finland have published several reports on the use of an *uncooked* vegan diet for RA (Hanninen et al., 2000). An uncooked vegan diet consists of vegetables, roots, nuts, germinated seeds, sprouts, cereals, fruits, and berries. This diet is often called a *"living food* diet." It is high in fiber, carotenoids, flavonoids, vitamins C and E, lycopen, and lutein. Some foods included in the diet are fermented and contain living lactobacilli, a bacterium which may have health benefits. Rheumatoid arthritis patients on this diet were reported to have improvement in symptoms as well as improvement in objective measures of their disease.

There are other small studies that show that vegetarian diets can reduce the signs and symptoms of RA. In a small but intensive Norwegian study (Kjeldsen-Kragh et al., 1991) a fasting diet consisting of vegetable juice was followed by a vegan and gluten-free diet. After three to five months, the experimental group progressed to a lactovegetarian diet for the remainder of the year. The study group participants noted improvement in arthritic symptoms compared to people on a well-balanced diet without restriction. Blood tests that indicate inflammation (see CRP and ESR, Chapter 3) showed reduced inflammation in the vegetarian group (Kjeldsen-Kragh et al., 1995a). It is not clear if the benefit comes from eliminating animal-derived products or from increasing fruits and vegetables. Some researchers hypothesize that meat is a major factor contributing to the inflammation of RA (Grant, 2000). However, plants are rich natural sources of vitamins, minerals, and antioxidants, and these nutrients might explain the benefit of this approach. There is a third hypothesis. Interestingly, in the Norwegian study, the vegetarians had less evidence of antibodies against the bacteria *Proteus mirabilis.* This raises the possibility that the improvement in RA activity may be related to the effects of the vegan diet on gut bacteria and the body's reaction to its presence (Kjeldsen-Kragh et al., 1995b; Kjeldsen-Kragh, 1999). Larger and better controlled studies are needed to answer these questions.

Since eliminating animal products can seriously decrease protein intake, you should work with a nutritionist or dietitian if you wish to do this. Professional nutritionists can help you plan meals that meet your daily requirements, particularly of amino acids, B vitamins, iron, and calcium. Remember that good muscle health is critical to properly functioning joints, and your muscles require essential amino acids, which are the building blocks of protein and muscle.

Gluten-Free Diet

The protein portion of wheat and closely related grains is termed **gluten.** People can be physically intolerant of wheat, and also of barley, oats, or rye. People with serious intolerance can develop a bowel problem called celiac disease. In addition, in some people, fatigue, nutrient deficiency, and achiness may be attributable to consumption of gluten.

In one study (Hafstrom et al., 2001), researchers showed that levels of antibodies against gliadin (a gluten protein) decreased in the group of patients with RA who had a good response to a gluten-free vegetarian diet. This suggests that *some* patients with RA may derive some benefit from a gluten-free diet. If this is an area of interest for you, there are blood tests that can be done to determine if you are sensitive to gluten. The two most common tests are *anti-gliadin antibodies* and *anti-endomysial antibody*. These antibodies can be elevated in some people with RA without causing bowel problems. At this time the significance of these antibodies is unclear. Gluten-restricted diets are difficult to maintain; the guidance of your doctor and possibly a dietitian are advised.

Fad Diets

Around every corner is a new diet that boasts weight loss and numerous health benefits. Suffice it to say that in most instances the science does not equal the hype. Some of these diets may even be dangerous for you. In most circumstances, we recommend that you follow the guidelines of a nutritious diet described above, and discuss variations to this with a certified health professional.

A Word on Food Supplements

Scientists are becoming increasingly interested in using food supplements as adjuncts to standard medication, and consumer interest in food supplements has exploded in the past decade. This interest was supported in Congress by the passage of the Dietary Supplement Health and Education Act of 1994 (DSHEA). This removed regulatory barriers that were said to be "limiting or slowing the flow of safe products and accurate information to consumers." As you have seen when reading magazines or watching television, this has allowed the supplement industry considerable leeway in making vague claims about effectiveness. The theory was that "consumers should be empowered to make choices about preventive health care programs based on data from scientific studies of health benefits related to particular dietary supplements." The Food and Drug Administration (FDA) regulates safety, manufacturing, and labeling, while the Federal Trade Commission (FTC) has jurisdiction over advertising claims for food supplements, under its consumer protection function.

A very important part of the DSHEA, however, has not been fully implemented. This is the section on strict manufacturing requirements, commonly called good manufacturing practices (GMPs). This allows the FDA to require that dietary supplements meet GMPs of potency, cleanliness, and stability. Unfortunately, at the time of this writing, the criteria are not being measured or monitored by anyone except the manufacturer. Amounts of active ingredients can still vary considerably between brands. There is little monitoring of additives, dyes, or contaminants. The FDA does not have to review or approve supplement ingredients or products before they are marketed. Currently, it is only *after* injury or harm to consumers has been proved that the FDA can use its authority and resources to remove a supplement from the market.

Many physicians are reluctant to consider or even discuss any form of food supplementation, because of lack of quality control regulations, the scarcity of research studies, the potential for harm, and the possibility of drug interactions. If your doctor is not interested and you have a strong wish to pursue this avenue, you may need to negotiate with your doctor. *Above all, do not take a supplement and hide the fact from your doctor.* It may be dangerous for your health and will certainly be harmful to a trusting doctor-patient relationship. You may never receive your doctor's "endorsement" of a supplement, but he or she needs to be informed should any negative effects occur.

Despite lack of scientific evidence, America has spoken. Food supplements constitute a multibillion-dollar business simply because they offer hope to many with chronic conditions. Fortunately, some supplements do hold promise for relief for arthritis symptoms, but we must overcome the quality control problems and get confirmatory evidence of effectiveness and safety. As a consequence of these circumstances, the number of funded studies for research on food supplements has increased markedly in the past decade.

Guidelines for Evaluating Food Supplements

Until science catches up to demand and regulation of supplements improves, patients are taking supplements at their own risk. There are some general principles that will help you lessen, but not remove, these risks. Here are some basic strategies to consider when making decisions about supplements.

When purchasing supplements:

· Consider only products from large companies, pharmacies, or reputable health food stores.
· Be cautious with Internet, mail order, magazine, or "infomercial" purchases unless the brands are well known.
· Look for ingredients with the U.S.P. notation, which indicates that the manufacturer has followed standards established by the U.S. Pharmacopoeia.

Make certain that the label of the supplement contains:

· Serving size
· Name and amount of active ingredient
· Name and place of manufacturer, packer, or distributor
· Directions for use

Avoid products offering or claiming:

· "Secret" ingredients
· A "cure," "breakthrough," or "new discovery"
· Only personal testimonials (patient stories) to show effectiveness
· A "quick fix" for chronic problems
· "Cure alls": claims to improve a wide range of unrelated problems
· To be "scientifically proven" but provides no references
· No side effects (even placebos have side effects)
· To "detoxify" or "purify"
· Wisdom of the ages as proof of safety: "time tested," "ancient remedies"

Always discuss with your physician any product you are considering using. Review with your doctor or pharmacist any potential drug interactions between the product you are considering taking and medications you are already taking.

As with any medicine, try only one new supplement at a time, to accurately determine benefit or side effects. Keep a record of the brand, the dose, and the time when you take it. *Never* take a greater amount than the label recommends. You *can* overdose on supplements.

Vitamins and Minerals

As mentioned above in the section on a well-balanced, nutritious diet, vitamins and minerals are critical to health. As much as possible, the recommended daily nutrients should be consumed through diet. When a busy life-style makes it difficult to eat a well-rounded diet, we often recommend that patients take a high-quality high-potency daily multivitamin with minerals that includes extra B vitamins and antioxidants. Low-quality vitamins may contain the right amounts of nutrients, but the nutrients may not be adequately absorbable, especially minerals, which are difficult to absorb in their original form. High-quality daily vitamin and mineral supplements often contain "chelated" minerals, which are more easily absorbed by the body. If you take more than one supplement, be certain to add up the individual vitamins and minerals from each supplement to avoid exceeding daily maximum amounts. This is particularly important with fat-soluble vitamins, which can accumulate in the body and cause toxicity. Don't forget to count the nutrients contained in drinks and shakes that are fortified with extra vitamins and minerals.

Many vitamins and minerals have been scrutinized to determine whether they could help in the treatment of rheumatoid arthritis. Reported vitamin and mineral deficiencies in people with RA have included deficiencies in vitamins C, D, B5, B6, B12, E, and folic acid, calcium, magnesium, zinc, and selenium. There is a growing scientific rationale for the use of dietary supplements as *adjuncts* in the treatment of inflammatory disorders like RA (Darlington, 2001). However, *no vitamin or mineral supplement has been proven to reduce the risk of structural damage that can be caused by rheumatoid arthritis.*

Vitamins

Vitamin A

Vitamin A is a fat-soluble vitamin with antioxidant properties. Its plant-derived precursor is beta carotene. Because vitamin A is required for normal immune system function, there is some potential value for people with RA. A Johns Hopkins study showed low levels of beta carotene and retinol, as well as vitamin E, in some people with RA (Comstock et al., 1997). There have been no studies demonstrating benefit of vitamin A supplementation for RA, however. Vitamin A is toxic in high doses. Beta carotene overdose is less common. It is best to get this vitamin from your diet. Foods high in vitamin A include fortified milk, leafy vegetables, sweet potatoes, carrots, and apricots.

B Vitamins

Water-soluble B vitamins include thiamin (B1), riboflavin (B2), niacin (B3), pantothenic acid (B5), pyridoxine (B6), cyanocobalamin (B12). A 1960s study showed people with RA to be partially deficient in B5

(Barton-Wright et al., 1963). Another small study showed some reduction in symptoms of RA after supplementation with B5 (General Practitioner Research Group, 1980). Good food sources for vitamin B5 are soybeans, lentils, eggs, grains, and meat.

Low levels of vitamin B6 have been noted in people with RA, particularly those with significant inflammation (Roubenoff et al., 1997). Some researchers have suggested that vitamin B6 is utilized in greater amounts when inflammation is present. Low B6 may also be linked to heart disease. This may account for the increased risk of cardiovascular disease that has been described with RA.

Vitamin B12 is important for the development of new red blood cells. Anemia can be a problem in people with RA, so getting adequate amounts of B12 is crucial, particularly when taking the medication methotrexate. Leafy green vegetables, legumes, peanuts, sunflower seeds, whole grains, meat, fish, and dairy products all contain B12. Again, we recommend taking a multivitamin with extra B vitamins.

Vitamin C

Vitamin C is a water-soluble antioxidant. As such, it may have benefits for inflammation. Citrus fruits (oranges, grapefruit, strawberries) and most vegetables (broccoli, red peppers, green peppers) are high in vitamin C.

Vitamin D

Vitamin D is a fat-soluble vitamin that is required for calcium absorption by the body. Some very early research suggests it may have a protective role in RA (Deluca and Cantoma, 2001). Vitamin D clearly is important for the prevention and treatment of osteoporosis, which can occur in RA (see Chapter 16 for more on preventing and treating osteoporosis). A typical multivitamin will contain 400 IU (international units) of vitamin D per day. Recommended doses in adults with RA are 400–800 IU per day. (Any postmenopausal woman with RA should take 800 IU, unless her doctor says otherwise.) Foods high in vitamin D include fortified milk and cold water fish, such as salmon, sardines, mackerel, herring, anchovy, and lake trout.

Vitamin E

Vitamin E is a major antioxidant, probably the most important in the body. It is crucial for maintaining a normal immune system. A small study showed low levels of vitamin E in inflamed rheumatoid joints (Fairburn et al., 1992), and other research indicated low amounts of vitamin E in the blood (Kajanachumpol et al., 2000). And several studies have suggested that people with RA may not be consuming enough vitamin E. Vitamin E supplementation has been reported to have some benefit for symptoms of RA in several small studies, the most recent in Egypt (Helmy et al., 2001). Larger studies are needed to verify these promising results.

Care should be exercised not to exceed the maximum dose of vitamin E. High doses can interfere with natural blood clotting and can interfere with the blood thinner Coumadin (warfarin). A recent study (Brown et al., 2001) suggested that supplemental vitamin E may blunt the beneficial effects of some cholesterol-lowering drugs. Foods naturally high in vitamin E include whole grains, nuts, seeds, poultry, and fish.

Folic Acid

Like vitamin B12, folate or folic acid is important for red blood cell development. It also helps lower homocysteine, high levels of which are linked to heart disease. Researchers at Tufts University have discovered that patients with RA appear to have increased risk of heart disease and increased homocysteine levels (Roubenoff et al., 1997). A diet rich in folic acid is recommended. Most multivitamins include folic acid. Daily recommendations are 200 micrograms per day. Foods high in folic acid include leafy green vegetables, legumes, broccoli, and dried beans.

Minerals

Boron

In one small study (Travers et al., 1990), researchers demonstrated that boron supplements relieved some of the symptoms of RA. We do not advise supplementation beyond the amount contained in a regular multivitamin with minerals. People with kidney problems should definitely avoid extra supplementation. Food sources include fruits, vegetables, nuts, and dried beans.

Calcium

Adequate calcium intake is critical to prevention of the bone loss associated with RA. (See Chapter 16 for details on calcium supplementation.)

Copper

Reports suggest that some people with RA are deficient in copper (DiSilvestro et al., 1992), but there is *no* evidence that oral supplementation with copper can help treat or slow RA. Many people advocate wearing copper bracelets and believe that trace amounts of copper are absorbed by a process called "dermal assimilation." One small study (Walker and Keats, 1976) did report positive results. Wearing copper is a benign treatment that the authors have no objection to. Foods high in copper include dried beans, shellfish, nuts, seeds, whole grains, vegetables, and chocolate. Supplementation of daily diet beyond a multivitamin with minerals is not recommended.

Selenium

Selenium is an essential trace mineral in the body. Plant foods are the major dietary source of selenium. Studies have indicated a low level of the antioxidant selenium in some people with severe RA (Tarp, 1995). Finnish studies suggest that low selenium and low vitamin E levels may be a risk factor for *developing* RA (Knekt et al., 2000). Studies disagree on the therapeutic value of selenium supplementation for people who have RA. We need further study to determine if there is any benefit to selenium supplementation. For now, until we have more evidence about using selenium for RA symptoms, it is best simply to make certain that your multivitamin contains selenium. Food sources of selenium include crab, liver, fish, Brazil nuts, and poultry.

Zinc

Zinc levels have been shown to be low in some people with RA. Studies have not indicated definitively whether or not supplementation provides benefit. Foods high in zinc include seafood, meats, egg yolk, whole grains, and legumes. If you take a multivitamin, it seems prudent to take one that includes zinc.

Herbs and Plant-Based Medicine

Many standard pharmaceutical medications are derived from plants. Their manufacture and standardization are carefully monitored and they must meet strict regulations. Unlike pharmaceutical drugs, medicinal herbal preparations are not necessarily produced with careful attention to standardization and quality control. Many people believe that herbs cannot be harmful because they are "natural." But, just as medicinal herbs can have good effects, they can also have bad effects. For all intents and purposes, herbs are medicines that do not have to pass the rigorous guidelines established by the Food and Drug Administration for effectiveness or safety.

With the current flurry of interest in herbal medicine, many companies are manufacturing these products. Some are legitimate high-quality herb manufacturers, but others use processing techniques that include additives, or use parts of the plant that are not proven to be therapeutic. Cases of contamination have particularly been a problem with Chinese and Ayurvedic herbs, requiring the removal of tainted products from the market. Contaminants, additives, and improper handling or storage will remain a concern until the FDA gains regulatory oversight of this industry and good manufacturing procedures (GMPs) can be enforced.

We are all optimistic about the prospect of safer natural remedies. Although there are exciting new studies about herbs and health, the authors suggest that you *avoid herbs for the treatment of RA*. We have two reasons for this advice. First, very little is known about drug interactions with other rheumatoid medications. Second, treatment for RA requires several different types of medications, and adding to that complexity may confuse the picture considerably if a side effect does occur.

The herbs discussed in this section are commonly advertised for the treatment of RA. *There is very little research to support their use in treating RA.*

Boswellia

Boswellia (*Boswellia serrata*) is an herb that has been used for centuries in Ayurvedic medicine (traditional medicine from India). It is regarded as anti-inflammatory. There is very little research regarding this herb and its use in treatment of RA.

Bromelain

Bromelain is an extract of the pineapple plant. Studies reveal that this plant enzyme has anti-inflammatory effects. It is commonly used in Germany to reduce swelling after injury. Its benefit in RA has not been proven. One small study (Cohen et al., 1964) suggested that bromelain might help reduce swelling and impaired joint mobility. Bromelain can also thin the blood and therefore may have the potential for a *drug interaction* with Coumadin (warfarin), heparin, and possibly with aspirin and NSAIDs. There is also a possibility of interaction with tetracycline antibiotics. Clearly, if you are taking minocycline for RA you should *avoid* this herb.

Cat's Claw

Cat's claw (*Uncaria tomentosa*) is made from the bark of a Peruvian vine. Although it is frequently used to treat RA, studies of its effectiveness have not been performed. Cat's claw has the potential for *drug interactions* with blood thinners such as Coumadin (warfarin) and heparin.

Chinese Herbs

The list of ancient Chinese herbs is lengthy. Many combinations are used. Unlike "Western herbs," Chinese herbs are often difficult for the lay person and even physicians to understand. In the United States, there are concerns about the lack of standardization and quality control. Herbal preparations tainted with aristocholic acid, a possible kidney carcinogen, recently were discovered. The result was an FDA-ordered recall and an increase in our concern about purity. If you must try these preparations, please purchase the herbs from a certified practitioner or an acupuncturist who is experienced and certified and who has a longstanding commitment to your community. Committed professionals would be more likely to use high-quality herbs from a reputable source and to help you determine if there are potential negative interactions with other medicines you are taking. Always inform your physician of these treatments.

Curcumin

Curcumin, an extract of the spice turmeric, has also been used for many years in Ayurvedic medicine. In the 1970s and 1980s Indian researchers confirmed its mild anti-inflammatory effects. Curcumin also appears to have antioxidant properties. This herb is widely used in India for RA. Because curcumin can cause gallbladder contraction, its use should be approved by your physician, particularly if you have gallbladder problems.

Devil's Claw

Devil's claw (*Harpagophytum procumbens*) comes from the root of an African plant. It is used in Europe as an anti-inflammatory treatment for rheumatoid arthritis. Although this herb is commonly used, there is no direct proof of its benefit for RA. It may cause a *drug interaction* with the blood thinner Coumadin (warfarin).

Feverfew

This herb has been used for many years to treat headaches and arthritis. Although there is some evidence of its benefit for migraines, there is no confirmation of its effectiveness in treating RA. A potential *drug interaction*: use of feverfew with NSAIDs might increase NSAID side effects such as stomach and kidney problems.

Ginger

Ginger is a common spice used in tea, soda, and food, and has long been employed medicinally. In at least Ayurvedic and Chinese herbal traditions it has been used for inflammation. Its benefit for RA has not been definitively proven. In large amounts, it may irritate the stomach, and may interact adversely with blood thinners.

Yucca

Yucca is commonly recommended for arthritis. However, there is no documented evidence of its effectiveness in RA.

Other Supplements

Glucosamine Sulfate and Chondroitin Sulfate

Glucosamine and chondroitin are substances that occur naturally in the body, manufactured versions of which have become part of mainstream medicine. Their popularity was ignited in part by a book titled *The Arthritis Cure*. The combination of glucosamine and chondroitin is frequently recommended by physicians for treatment of osteoarthritis. Formal studies have demonstrated some symptom relief for patients with *osteoarthritis* (degenerative arthritis). The effectiveness of these supplements lies in their benefit to cartilage that has been broken down by the forces of wear and tear. Unfortunately, these supplements have not been shown to help with the symptoms or progress of rheumatoid arthritis. This is almost certainly because the damage from RA comes from inflammation and not from wear and tear. These two supplements do not directly affect inflammation in a meaningful way.

Essential Fatty Acids: EPA, DHA, and GLA

We read every day about the benefits of reducing fat in our diets. Saturated oils, particularly from red meat, are clearly associated with harmful effects on total cholesterol and on the heart. Unsaturated fatty acids, however, are essential for good health. In fact, some essential fatty acids have anti-inflammatory effects and may help patients with RA. There are two families of essential fatty acids: omega-3 and omega-6. Omega-3 fatty acids are present in certain fish and plant seeds. Two omega-3 fatty acids, eicosapentaenoic acid (EPA) and docosahexaenoic acid (DHA), both found in fish oil, have been studied most closely; they show anti-inflammatory effects with RA. Flaxseed oil is high in a fatty acid called alpha-linolenic acid (AL), which our bodies can convert to EPA. ALA may be helpful but is not as well studied and may not be as potent as EPA and DHA.

Some vegetable oils have high amounts of omega-6 fatty acids. When balanced with omega-3 fatty acids, they also promote good health. However, if consumed in amounts *exceeding* the intake of omega-3 fatty acids, they may actually fuel inflammation. Oils with mostly omega-6 fatty acids include corn oil, sunflower oil, and safflower oil. These oils are taken in overabundance in the American diet. Oils with a more healthful balance of omega-3 as compared to omega-6 fatty acids are olive oil, flaxseed oil, or canola oil. A 1999 Harvard study looked at the benefits of the Mediterranean diet in Greek patients. They found that patients who consumed more olive oil and more vegetables were less likely to develop RA (Linos et al., 1999). Trying to improve the omega-3 over omega-6 balance appears to be a worthy endeavor.

Contrary to the above observation, there are certain omega-6 fatty acid derivatives that may help inflammation. Gamma-linolenic acid (GLA) is an essential fatty acid found in evening primrose oil, borage oil, and black currant oil. There is early evidence that GLA may help RA symptoms, and more promising studies are underway (Zurier et al., 1996). Be careful about GLA supplements; they can have *drug interactions* with blood thinners.

Fish Oil

Fish oil treatment for RA has been more rigorously studied than any other natural remedy. Several studies have determined that fish oil supplementation can reduce the pain and swelling of RA. The most influential of the published studies are being led by Joel Kremer at the Albany (New York) Medical Center. The omega-3 fatty acids in fish oil are thought to be responsible for its anti-inflammatory effects. The two most important fatty acids are EPA and DHA (see above). Supplements of these substances have been shown to reduce both the number of swollen joints and morning stiffness (Kremer, 2000). There is currently no evidence that fish oil treatment has any advantage over **NSAIDs** or that it slows the progression of RA, as **DMARDs** do.

Not all fish oils are equal. Cod liver oil, for example, is very high in vitamin A and vitamin D as well as omega-3 fatty acids. These fat-soluble vitamins can build up in your body and cause toxic effects; therefore, you should keep track of the content of fat-soluble vitamins in all supplements you take. Other possible complications include bloating, gas, and short-term increase in LDL, or "bad" cholesterol. Fish oil also has blood thinning characteristics. This may present a potential *drug interaction* when combined with an anticoagulant medication (prescription blood thinner) such as Coumadin (warfarin) or heparin. In people at risk for bleeding, combining fish oil with aspirin or NSAIDs may not be advisable. Always ask your doctor.

The safest way to get the value of fish oils is to increase the amount of fresh cold water fish in your diet. Cold water fish include sardines, salmon, mackerel, herring, anchovy, and lake trout.

For More Information

The Arthritis Foundation offers *Diet and Your Arthritis* and the "2001 Supplement Guide," which will likely be updated and is available in printed form and on the Arthritis Foundation Web site, with other valuable information, at *www.arthritis.org/conditions/SupplementGuide.*

The USDA posts updated information on "The Food Guide Pyramid" on its Web site, http://www.pueblo.gsa.gov.

Other governmental sources of information are:

Food and Nutrition Information Center, National Agricultural Library, USDA, 10301 Baltimore Blvd., Room 304, Beltsville, Md. 20705-2351; www.fns.usda.gov/fns

Healthfinder-Gateway to Reliable Consumer Health Information, U.S. Department of Health and Human Services, P.O. Box 1133, Washington, D.C. 20013-1133; www.healthfinder.gov

National Institutes of Health, Office of Dietary Supplements (ODS), Building 31, Room 1B25, 31 Center Drive, MSC 2086, Bethesda, Md. 20892-9663; 301-435-2920, fax 301-480-1845; http://dietary-supplements.info.nih.gov; and http://www.cc.nih.gov/ccc/supplements/intro.html

National Institutes of Health International Bibliographic Information on Dietary Supplements (IBIDS) database: http://ods.od.nih.gov/databases/ibids.html

U.S. Department of Agriculture, http://www.nal.usda.gov/fnic/IBIDS

Finally, the American Dietetic Association, 216 West Jackson Blvd., Suite 800, Chicago, Ill. 60606-6995, provides a consumer nutrition hotline, 1-800-366-1655, and a Web site, www.eatright.org.

CHAPTER 19

Surgery for Rheumatoid Arthritis

•

Sometimes, despite timely medical therapy, rheumatoid arthritis (RA) continues to cause inflammation and joint damage. When other therapies haven't been successful, surgery may be necessary. Surgical techniques are constantly being improved, providing new alternatives to help people with RA.

Surgery is recommended for a variety of reasons, the most common of which is to control severe pain caused by inflammation or damaged joints. Surgery may also be advised to repair ruptured ligaments or tendons or to remove inflamed synovial tissue that has not responded adequately to other therapy and which threatens to cause joint damage. Finally, surgery may be the recommended treatment to retain or restore function in a specific joint.

Some surgical procedures are intended to provide temporary relief and to prevent damage over the long term. Others are corrective measures aimed at improving the function of joints that have already been damaged.

Surgeons Specializing in the Treatment of RA

Your primary care doctor or **rheumatologist** may recommend that you have a consultation with a surgeon to determine whether a surgical procedure will help you. The specific problems you are having and the joints involved will to some extent determine the type of surgeon you see. The expertise of the surgeons practicing in your geographical area will also influence your choice.

Surgeons who specialize in performing surgery on bones and joints are called **orthopedic surgeons.** These professionals perform surgical procedures on the large joints such as the shoulders, elbows, hips, and knees. Many also have expertise in surgeries of the smaller joints of the hands and feet. Some orthopedic surgeons are experts in specific types of surgery, such as joint reconstruction or arthroscopic surgery.

Hand surgeons are generally highly specialized; most of them have training in either orthopedic surgery or **plastic surgery**. Often they will have obtained specialized training in surgery of the upper extremities. If they have had this formal fellowship training, they can be certified as hand subspecialists.

Podiatrists are specialists in the medical and surgical treatment of foot ailments. Many podiatrists perform surgery on the feet of people with RA. This is an area of expertise which they share with some orthopedic surgeons.

Types of Surgery

Some of the basic types of joint surgeries are discussed below. For an animated view of these surgeries, visit the Arthritis Foundation's on-line site Surgery Center, which presents surgery animations and provides other timely information (www.arthritis.org/conditions/SurgeryCenter).

Arthroscopic Surgery

By inserting a pencil-sized scope called an *arthroscope* through a small incision in the skin, a surgeon or rheumatologist is able to look inside the joint without putting the patient through major surgery. Being able to see the inside joint structures helps the surgeon determine what conditions are creating problems. While the surgeon is examining the inside of the joint, he or she can take a biopsy of tissue within the joint to confirm a diagnosis or perform simple corrective procedures, such as removing damaged **cartilage**.

More extensive surgical procedures such as ligament and tendon repairs can also be performed through an arthroscope. Arthroscopic synovectomy is another common procedure.

Synovectomy

Synovectomy is the name of the procedure in which the effects of destructive **synovitis** are removed. Inflamed joint lining (**synovium**) is removed surgically to prevent it from damaging cartilage and other joint structures. Although very effective in reducing joint pain and swelling, synovectomy should not be viewed as providing a permanent cure, because the synovium can grow back, and complete removal of all synovial tissue is not possible.

Synovectomy can be performed through an arthroscope. This approach has an advantage over open surgical synovectomy in that it avoids cutting and opening the joint capsule. For this reason, recovery from arthroscopic synovectomy is generally quite rapid.

Although it is more invasive, an open surgical synovectomy also has certain advantages. It provides the surgeon a better view of, and improved access into, the total joint, thereby facilitating thorough removal of the inflamed synovial tissue.

Synovectomies are frequently performed in the wrist, elbows, and knees. This surgery is often combined with tendon repair or reconstruction or with bone resection (see below).

Tendon Reconstruction and Transfers

RA can damage or even rupture surrounding tendons and ligaments. If the tendon is ruptured, it is possible to reconstruct the tendon by connecting a separate but intact tendon to the ruptured one. This procedure is known as *tendon transfer*. Rupture is most common in the tendons that travel along the top of the hands down to the fingers.

Joint Fusion

Joint fusion, or *arthrodesis,* is a surgical procedure that permits bone to be connected to bone across a joint. This procedure is performed only on painful and unstable joints, most commonly in the wrists, feet, ankles, and thumbs. It very effectively decreases pain and improves stability, but it permanently inhibits motion in the fused joint. For this reason, joint fusion is rarely performed on the shoulder or hip.

With longstanding RA involving the neck, the vertebrae can become unstable because of ligament and bone loss caused by the synovitis. In severe cases, an operation to fuse the vertebrae may be required to increase stability.

Osteotomy and Bone Resection

Osteotomy is a procedure that involves cutting and repositioning the bone to improve joint alignment and to compensate for deformity. This procedure is performed less frequently than it once was, because improved joint replacement procedures provide more effective treatment.

Sometimes a section of bone is removed (*resected*) from the end nearest the joint. This form of bone resection is a simple procedure and is performed on joints in the shoulders, elbows, wrists, and feet to improve the joint's range of motion and to relieve pain.

Joint Replacement

New techniques of joint replacement, or *arthroplasty,* have dramatically improved the outlook for people with RA. In arthroplasty, a severely damaged joint is reconstructed. This may involve only resurfacing the damaged ends of bones on either side and realignment of the joint, or it may involve replacing the entire damaged joint with an artificial one.

In the past, total joint replacement was performed only in older, inactive individuals who had less chance of wearing out their new joints. However, current trends in surgery reflect the opinion that preserving function is mandatory for good health, and therefore the use of artificial joints in younger, more active individuals has increased. Total joint replacement is frequently performed in the knees, hips, and shoulders, with excellent results. Replacements for the elbows, wrists, and ankles are available, but the outcome is not as predictable. New designs are continually becoming available, however, and will likely provide better and more consistent results.

Artificial joints can be attached to the bone by two different methods. In the first, surgeons insert the stem of the replacement joint into a hole drilled into the bone; the hole is filled with a special cementing material called methylmethacrylate. This method is less painful and facilitates rehabilitation with faster healing, but the cement may crack and the joint may loosen in time, particularly in very active individuals.

Recently, surgeons have begun utilizing cementless joint replacements, the second method of attaching the artificial joint to the bone. In this method, the replacement stem, which has small pores in it, is inserted snugly into a perfectly matched hole in the bone. The patient's own bone slowly grows into the pores to provide stability. If successful, this method of replacement has the benefits of increased strength and durability, with (theoretically) a decreased need for additional replacement surgery in the future. Its disadvantages include prolonged rehabilitation and potential problems with delayed healing, as well as bone growth inadequate to support and stabilize the replacement. This bone growth inadequacy may be more likely to occur in individuals with RA whose bones have already been weakened by arthritis and some medications.

Joint replacements do not last forever, which is why many doctors favor postponing replacement until it becomes absolutely necessary. The newer techniques and materials have increased the life of a replacement joint to 15 years or more, under good conditions. Efforts to prolong the life of the replacement with joint protection measures such as weight management are very important. If the replacement breaks down, *revision arthroplasty* is often very successful.

Preparing for and Recovering from Surgery

Before Surgery

Be certain that your *surgeon* is aware of *all* of the medications you are taking, particularly nonsteroidal anti-inflammatory drugs (**NSAIDs**), immunosuppressants, corticosteroids, and **biologic response modifiers**. Remember to mention over-the-counter medications, such as ibuprofen or aspirin, and herbal preparations. To reduce the risk of excessive bleeding, NSAIDs are generally discontinued before surgery. Because surgery can lead to higher than normal risk for infection, medications that can inhibit or suppress the immune system are generally stopped for a short time before and after surgery. This would include medications such as methotrexate, cyclosporine, Enbrel, and Kineret. Make sure that you discuss your medications with *both* your prescribing physician and your surgeon when you are making plans for surgery.

If you are scheduled to have general anesthesia, tell your surgeon about any history of neck or jaw discomfort. Some surgeons request that a neck x-ray be taken in individuals who have had RA a long time. These precautions are often taken before general anesthesia is administered.

Before you undergo any joint replacement surgery, make certain that your orthopedic surgeon is aware of *any* infections you have, including skin breakdown and bladder infections. It is possible for infection to spread to the new joint by way of the bloodstream, so your surgeon will want to treat the infection if possible before proceeding. A common problem that people neglect to mention to their surgeon is severe dental caries (cavities) or tooth decay. Whether or not you have tooth decay, scrupulous dental hygiene is essential after a joint replacement, to avoid spreading bacteria into the new joint.

Ask your physician well in advance of the surgery whether it is possible for you to put aside your own blood in case you need blood during the procedure. Receiving your own blood is called an *autologous transfusion* and is the safest kind. The medication *erythropoietin* can be administered to people with **anemia** to stimulate the production of red blood cells; this should make it possible for someone with anemia to put blood aside in advance in case it is needed during surgery.

Before having surgery, do some home planning. Think about preparing meals ahead and freezing them. Arrange for help with everyday tasks in advance so you will be prepared after surgery. Rearrange furniture and equipment so you can get to what you need easily and safely. Too many people only consider these issues after the surgery is performed. *Plan ahead.*

During Your Recovery

You can increase the extent and speed of your recovery by actively participating in rehabilitation both before and after surgery, so the best advice we can give you is to follow the instructions of your **physical** and **occupational therapists** closely. Also, be certain to discuss with your orthopedic surgeon any exercise program involving a joint that has been operated on. Speak with your doctors about restarting any medications that have been temporarily discontinued.

For More Information

Order a copy of "Surgery and Arthritis: What You Need to Know," a free pamphlet from the Arthritis Foundation. Also visit www.arthritis.org/ resources for the "Surgery Center," which has very useful and specific surgical information.

PART VI

Practical Matters

•

Disability, Insurance, and Other Financial Matters

•

There's no getting around the fact that rheumatoid arthritis (RA) can interfere with a person's ability to work. Stiffness, pain, decreased mobility, and fatigue present problems for someone whose employment involves an eight-hour or longer workday. Since the passage of the *Americans with Disabilities Act (ADA)* in 1990, most employers are required by law to make reasonable accommodations to help employees keep working. We have already mentioned that people with RA often find it helpful to talk with their employers about arranging for increased flexibility in work hours and creating an arthritis-friendly workplace. These modifications can help a person with RA avoid interference with work because of minor flare-ups. Another possibility is a job-sharing program, in which two people each work half-time to fulfill the duties of one full-time job.

We stress the fact that persons with RA are *differently abled* and that, with creative planning, flexibility, and understanding, a person with RA often can continue in his or her job. This is what many people would prefer to do; but sometimes, despite a person's best creative efforts, it is not possible to continue being employed as before. This is particularly true for people with a physically demanding job that requires repeated use of inflamed joints.

A person with RA who is having problems at work would be well advised to discuss the situation with his or her doctor and a social service worker. If the best decision seems to be to make a change, the person might consider pursuing another form of employment, making arrangements with his or her employer to change jobs within the same company (or to change the description and duties of the present job), or applying for disability benefits. This decision, of course, is highly personal. The choice you make depends on your work experience, education, age, financial responsibilities, degree of arthritis involvement, and the advice of your health care team.

Disability Benefits

Should you decide to stop working, you may be eligible for disability benefits. These benefits vary greatly depending on the coverage offered by your employer and the availability of benefits for which you may be eligible. The definition of *disability* varies considerably among benefit providers, too. The following kinds of disability benefits may be available to you.

Commercial and Employment Disability Programs

Some companies offer short-term or long-term disability insurance as part of a benefits package. If disability insurance is an *optional* benefit in which you have chosen to participate, premium payments may be deducted from your paycheck. Disability benefits are often available for military or civil service employees.

Some people purchase individual disability policies from private insurance companies. Before signing up for disability insurance, read the insurance contract carefully to determine how long you need to be disabled before benefits begin and how *disability* is defined. Some policies are quite restrictive in these regards and may not be worth the investment.

State Disability Policies

Some states have disability insurance programs. People enrolled in these programs contribute a portion of the premium by way of a payroll deduction. Benefits are generally paid in proportion to the amount contributed to the fund. Your doctor will be familiar with your state's disability benefits and can tell you how to join the program.

Social Security Disability Benefits

You may be eligible for federal benefit programs if you are disabled by your arthritis. The definition of *disability* is based on your present and projected inability to perform *any* kind of work. You may be considered disabled by Social Security standards if:

· your arthritis prevents you from being gainfully employed and
· your condition is expected to last for at least one year or to result in death.

Social Security officers review your history, medical records, and personal physician's reports to determine whether you are disabled. A physical examination by a consulting physician may be requested by the agency if additional information about your current physical condition is needed. The reviewers will determine whether your arthritis matches disability standards set forth by an objective *listing of impairments.*

According to Social Security regulations, to qualify as having disabling RA, a person must show proof of persistent joint pain, swelling, or tenderness in multiple joints. Signs of joint inflammation (swelling and tenderness) must have been present for at least three months despite therapy and must have resulted in decreased function of those joints. It must be expected that the arthritis will remain a physical impairment for longer than twelve months. The results of such RA laboratory tests as **ESR** (erythrocyte sedimentation rate), **rheumatoid factor,** ANA (antinuclear antibody), and biopsy (see Chapter 3) must also be recorded as abnormal. Other factors taken into consideration include pain, fatigue, ability to perform basic work-related activities, age, education, past work experience, and transferable skills. The process of determining eligibility for benefits may take several months to complete. It is a good idea to keep in touch with the Social Security office during this time to monitor the progress being made on your case.

The Social Security Administration offers two disability programs, the Disability Insurance (DI) program and the Supplemental Security Income (SSI) program. Rules regarding eligibility for the two differ. DI benefits are based on work history, while SSI is based on financial need. Neither of these programs is designed to cover short-term or partial disability, as some private policies do.

Disability Insurance (DI). These Social Security benefits are funded through FICA taxes paid by both employees and employers. You may be eligible if you meet the disability standards described above. You and certain members of your family may qualify for DI if, in addition:

· you have sufficient work credits (determined by your length of employment, how recently you have worked, and the age at which you became disabled) or
· you are not engaged in substantial gainful activity (in 2002, this was defined as not having earnings of more than $780 per month on average).

Benefits usually begin after six full months of disability. The amount of your monthly disability benefit is based upon your lifetime average earnings covered by Social Security. You can obtain an estimate of your disability benefit from a Social Security office. Ask for a Social Security statement that displays your earning record and provides an estimate of your disability benefit. Payments are larger for people with dependents. Benefits may be adjusted if you are eligible for other federal disability benefits or for state, civil service, or military disability benefits. After twenty-four months of receiving DI, an individual qualifies for Medicare insurance.

Supplemental Security Income (SSI). This program is funded through general revenue funds. Again, to receive SSI benefits, you must be qualified as disabled according to the Social Security standards mentioned above. Unlike for DI, to be eligible for SSI you do not have to have a work history; instead, you must prove financial need, sufficient limitation of income and resources.

In determining financial need, the Social Security office will take into consideration the income and assets of your spouse, if you are married. Not all income and resources are included in determining eligibility, however; a portion of your monthly income, the value of food stamps, and most home energy assistance funds are not counted as income. Your personal home as well as burial plots (and money saved for burial costs) do not count as resources. Automobiles and life insurance policies are generally not counted unless their value exceeds the limits set forth by SSI regulations.

You should apply at any Social Security office as soon as you become disabled. Before going to the office, be sure to call the toll-free number for the agency, in your telephone directory. Social Security staff will answer many of your questions, tell you what records and documents to have ready, and direct you to the nearest Social Security office. You can speed up the process by having all requested documents when you make application. The office will send your completed application to the Disability Determination Services (DDS) in your state. The DDS will review your medical history and available records. Occasionally, a further medical consultation is requested. Decisions regarding your claim will be sent to your home. If you are denied benefits, information on the appeal process will also be sent.

Benefits will begin immediately after your application has been approved. The length of time required to qualify varies considerably, depending on the nature of your disability, your needs, and the accessibility and complexity of your medical and financial information. The benefit amount varies from state to state. Medicaid benefits may or may not begin immediately upon SSI approval. Medicaid eligibility also varies from state to state (your local Social Security office will be able to provide you with information about benefits in your state).

The *Ticket to Work and Work Incentives Act of 1999* substantially expanded opportunities for people receiving Social Security benefits to return to work on a trial basis. These "work incentives" allow trial work periods while the person continues to receive cash benefits and Medicare coverage. This act has removed some difficult obstacles for the many people who wish to try to return to work. With the new treatments for RA, this has been a very valuable change in Social Security rules.

Vocational Rehabilitation Benefits

Vocational Rehabilitation (VR) is a program jointly funded by the federal and state governments which helps disabled individuals become employable. To be eligible for VR, your disability *must directly interfere with your ability to work.* Therefore, you must currently be unemployed to qualify. VR services include counseling, medical help, job training, educational opportunities, financial assistance, job placement, and on-the-job assistance.

If you are receiving Social Security benefits as a result of your disability, you may be automatically referred to VR. If you are not receiving DI or SSI, you may still qualify for VR in some states in which VR finances are available. The resources of each state differ markedly, because the funds available reflect contributions allocated to the program.

The district office for VR is listed under state government services in the telephone book.

Health Insurance

Private Health Insurance

If you are working and your employer provides health insurance benefits, you may not have the option of selecting a specific form of insurance or a specific insurance carrier. (*Note:* If you are insured through a group plan at work and then lose your job or begin to consider another job, *do not* drop your health insurance. More information on this is given below.)

If you do have a choice when it comes to health insurance, we recommend that you examine carefully several types of policies and look into several insurance carriers before making a decision. Choosing wisely is important, especially because it is sometimes difficult to make changes in insurance coverage if your health deteriorates in any way.

Selecting the best form of health insurance involves choosing among many variables. Asking the following key questions may help you choose wisely.

For standard policies:

· Is there a deductible? (And can you afford to pay that deductible each year?)
· Are there large co-payments? (If so, do lower premiums offset that expense?)

· What percentage of expenses are you responsible for after the deductible has been met? (Would you prefer to pay higher premiums in exchange for paying a lower percentage of a covered expense?)
· Is there a "cap" on the amount you have to pay, if a percentage payment applies? (For your protection, there should be.)

For a health maintenance organization (HMO) or prepaid medical insurance:

· Is your choice of physicians limited? If so, is there a **rheumatologist** and an **orthopedic surgeon** experienced in joint surgery on the *preferred provider* staff? (If the services of these specialists aren't provided, can you get the HMO or preferred insurance carrier to agree to pay for the services of such specialists if needed?)
· Are you permitted to use only specific hospitals and specific **physical therapy** services? (If so, find out—by asking your present doctor if necessary—whether the permitted service providers have a good reputation for treatment of RA.)
· Do the primary care doctors in the HMO readily refer their patients for specialty consultation? (They ought to.)

For all insurance:

· Does your policy cover **physical therapy, occupational therapy,** and the services of a **podiatrist?** (If not, you'll probably want to choose a different policy.)
· Is there a prescription policy? (We recommend that you enroll in an insurance plan that pays most of the cost of prescription drugs, because arthritis medications can be extremely costly.)
· Will your policy cover *durable medical equipment* such as splints, braces, orthotics, walking aids? (If there is an additional premium for this coverage, you'll have to decide whether you would prefer to pay the cost of these aids out of pocket as necessary or whether it is better for you to pay the additional premium on a regular basis.)
· Is there a *preexisting illness* clause that may limit payment for costs related to your RA? (If so, the wiser choice, if it is available, might be to pay a higher premium and obtain coverage for the preexisting condition.)

It is critical that you examine your insurance options if your employment status is about to change. Be very careful: because you have RA, you may run into difficulties in getting another insurance carrier to cover you. A federal law, COBRA (Consolidated Omnibus Budget Reconciliation Act) requires that employees, in most cases, be allowed to convert their group insurance into an individual policy that will be guaranteed at the group premium rate for a given time period. However, before you discontinue your coverage under your former employer's group plan—or allow your former employer to discontinue your coverage—be sure to review your new policy and be certain that it has gone into effect. You will have to pay the premium for this new insurance, of course.

While you are covered under COBRA, explore other options: can you obtain coverage under your spouse's policy, for example, or can you get group insurance through a new job or a professional society? Take every possible precaution to prevent a lapse in coverage. Our experience tells us that insurance carriers are often most reluctant to provide comprehensive coverage to people with chronic medical problems. This is why we emphasize the importance of holding on to one health insurance policy until another one has gone into effect.

Government Health Insurance

Medicare. People may qualify for this federally funded health insurance program if they are over age 65 *or* if they have received Social Security Disability Insurance for more than twenty-four months.

There are two parts of Medicare: Part A and Part B. Part A covers inpatient hospital care and is financed through FICA taxes. Part B covers a percentage of doctors' fees, x-rays, and diagnostic tests. This portion of Medicare is financed through monthly premiums paid by the individual.

Medicare insurance provides limited coverage. It does not pay for medications, for example. In addition, many physicians will not "*accept assignment*" (the amount that Medicare agrees a given service should cost) as full payment because this reimbursement is significantly less than the average fee charged by physicians. Medicare also requires the insured person to pay a significant deductible as well as an additional 20 percent of *approved* assignments. Consequently, it is wise to purchase a supplemental health insurance policy which will help pay the costs that Medicare does not cover. There are also many senior HMO insurance products that may be available in your community.

Medicaid. This health insurance is jointly funded by the federal and state governments and is available to individuals with low income. Disabled persons with low income may also be eligible. Most individuals who qualify for SSI will automatically qualify for Medicaid in most states. Other eligibility qualifications vary extensively among states, and these qualification criteria are constantly changing in response to the constantly escalating costs of health care.

Because the amount reimbursed to physicians from Medicaid is extremely limited, many physicians in private practice and HMOs hesitate to treat patients who have this form of health insurance. Federally funded clinics, hospitals, and university centers, however, will usually accept Medicaid insurance, especially if you reside in their region.

Veterans Administration (VA) Benefits

The VA offers both health care and disability help to veterans who qualify. Although all service-connected disabilities are covered by the VA, rheumatoid arthritis generally does not qualify as a service-connected disability, and so eligibility for treatment of RA would depend on other criteria, such as your income and ability to pay. The benefit specialist at the local VA center can assist you by outlining the options available to you. If you are a veteran, find out what benefits you are eligible to receive.

Income Taxes

Having RA can be quite expensive, especially with the advent of biologic response modifiers. For tax purposes, the question is whether your expenses in any one year are high enough to be tax deductible. Generally, medical and dental expenses are only deductible when they reach extremely high levels—currently, more than 7.5 percent of your adjusted gross income. If you spend a large amount of money for health care, however, you may be able to get some assistance in the form of a tax break. The tax code's definition of expenditures for medical care is amounts paid for the "diagnosis, cure, mitigation, treatment, or prevention of disease, and for treatments affecting any part or function of the body." Qualifying expenses may include capital expenditures for special equipment or for home improvements if their main purpose is medical care: building ramps; widening doors; changing counter heights or fixtures; installing railings, handrails, or grab bars; modifying hardware; and so on. Generally a doctor's order will suffice to qualify for a deduction of reasonable costs. Other deductible expenses are car modifications, chiropractic and dental care, medications, eyeglasses, trained animals for assistance, hearing aids, home care, health insurance premiums, *qualified* long-term care contracts, stop-smoking programs, and *physician-directed* weight loss programs.

Tax laws change continually, so you (and your accountant) will need to keep abreast of them. Currently, you can refer to the following Internal Revenue Service publications for information: 502 ("Medical and Dental Expenses"), 524 ("Credit for the Elderly or the Disabled"), and 907 ("Tax

Information for Persons with Handicaps or Disabilities"). To order these publications, call 1-800-TAX-FORM.

If your health care expenses are high but not high enough to be deductible on your income taxes, there may be other options. Many corporations offer a "cafeteria/flexible benefits" program (under section 125 of the Internal Revenue Code) which allows you to use *pretax* dollars to pay for your health costs. In this way, you do not pay income taxes on income that you spend on health care. Find out whether this program is available where you or your spouse works. If not, you may be able to promote some interest in the program in the personnel or human resources department.

Whatever your insurance or tax situation, save all of your receipts for any expenses that relate to your RA, including home modifications or special expenses that are a result of your arthritic condition.

For More Information

A free consulting agency, the Job Accommodation Network, operated by the President's Committee on Employment of People with Disabilities, provides information on the Americans with Disabilities Act (ADA) and types of accommodations. Telephone 1-800-526-7234.

For numerous publications and other information about Social Security benefits, contact your local Social Security office or write or call the national office: Social Security Administration, Office of Public Inquiries, 6401 Security Blvd., Baltimore, Md. 21235-6401; toll-free 1-800-772-1213, TTY 1-800-325-0778; Web site www.ssa.gov.

To contact Social Security for information about and help finding vocational rehabilitation, call toll-free 1-866-968-7842, TTY 1-866-833-2967.

Contact your local chapter or the national office of the Arthritis Foundation for copies of the free pamphlet "Arthritis and the Workplace."

About income taxes, IRS forms, and publications, write to: Internal Revenue Service, Technical Publications Branch, W:CAR:MP:FP:P, 1111 Constitution Ave. N.W., Washington, D.C. 20224; or call 1-800-TAX-FORM (1-800-829-3676). The Web site is www.irs.gov.

CHAPTER 21

Other Issues

•

Surfing the Net: Empowerment or Deception?

We have arrived conclusively in the information era. The Internet has allowed us to get up-to-date information in real time. It has given both patients and physicians access to resources that were not available in preceding decades. Universities, professional associations, legitimate advocacy groups, national public service programs, and not-for-profit organizations like the Arthritis Foundation provide valuable information on-line to people with RA. The abundance of resources is very exciting and has been long awaited by people looking for cutting-edge information. At the same time, the Internet is available to profiteers, pseudo-experts, and unqualified practitioners who prey on the pain and suffering of others. Many promoters pose as legitimate organizations or foundations in an effort to deceive people, making false promises in exchange for their victims' hard-earned money. You should avoid these sites and fight the understandable urge to try their products.

The Internet sites we list in this book present balanced information. Some of these sites are sponsored by the pharmaceutical industry; they promote products, but they also give great insight into RA. They are certainly worth investigating. However, keep in mind that they may reveal a bias toward the medication being marketed. We would also like to give you a few guidelines for choosing Internet sites as you surf the Web.

Consider sites that:

· represent organizations known to be legitimate, such as the Arthritis Foundation (remember that most legitimate "institutes," "foundations," and "associations" do *not* promote products)
· are associated with universities or medical centers
· are federally sponsored, such as those from the NIH, USDA, or FDA
· are recommended by legitimate authorities

Avoid sites that:

- are selling a specific therapy
- use "official" sounding but unfamiliar names (check out "Questionable Organizations: An Overview" at www.quackwatch.com
- do not list references for their "science" or "research"
- do not give an address (Post Office boxes do not count)
- do not give a telephone number to call if you want to ask questions
- accuse the medical profession and pharmaceutical companies of conspiracy
- oppose proven public health measures such as immunization or fluoridation

Clinical Research

What Is Clinical Research?

Exciting and promising new medications for the treatment of RA are around the corner. All new therapies must go through stringent testing and receive approval from the Food and Drug Administration (FDA) before they are made available to the public. Testing ensures that new treatments are both safe and effective. Clinical trials of new treatments are conducted by physicians in medical offices, hospitals, teaching universities, and research centers under the direction of a pharmaceutical company and the FDA. Clinical trials are generally conducted in three phases:

How Do Clinical Studies Operate?

Phase I

The first step in a clinical trial program for a new product candidate is a Phase I clinical trial. Phase I trials are designed to screen a substance for safety and to find the maximum safe dose.

Phase II

Phase II studies are undertaken to establish dosing and duration of treatment. Therapeutic effectiveness and safety are also evaluated.

Phase III

The final phase in a clinical study is designed to confirm effectiveness in larger patient populations and to continue monitoring for rare but significant side effects. Phase III trials are conducted in large groups of patients and generally compare the new product to another treatment.

Should I Participate in a Clinical Trial?

Participation in a clinical trial is completely voluntary. Before joining a study, a volunteer will receive an *informed consent* form, which should provide detailed information about the treatment, the potential side effects, the kind and number of visits that will be required, and any procedures that may be done. The physician and staff conducting the study should review with you any questions you have. They will also discuss treatment options that are *not* part of the research study, so you can understand the range of options available to you. Study participants have the right to *withdraw their consent at any time* during the study. The decision to participate in a clinical study is a very personal one. Volunteers are needed to bring these exciting new therapies to the public, and many people enjoy contributing to the research effort and having the opportunity to be the first to try a new therapy. On the other hand, many people prefer to wait until a therapy is fully tested. As always, your physician will help guide you in these decisions. Never let anyone pressure you into joining a study that you are not comfortable with.

Travel Tips

Sometimes people with RA give up vacation trips and other activities involving travel because they are afraid that they'll encounter insurmountable obstacles or barriers when they're away from home. Traveling is a wonderful pastime, though, and one you need not deny yourself. With careful planning, people with RA can travel almost wherever they choose.

Medical Tips for Travelers

Always discuss your vacation plans with your doctor. Ask him or her to recommend physicians where you are going who will consult with you and treat any unexpected problems that arise.

Take along one or two weeks' worth of medication *beyond* what you expect to need, as well as extra clearly written prescriptions from your doctor, in case your trip is prolonged unexpectedly.

Keep your medication separate from your luggage; that way, if your luggage is misplaced or stolen, you will still have your medication. It's best to keep your medication with you.

Carry a description of your medical problems and a list of your medications on your person. This information will be very useful if, in an emergency, you are unable to speak. Wearing a Medic Alert bracelet or necklace designating your medication allergies and other important medical information is a good idea. (For more information about acquiring a bracelet write: Medic Alert, Box 1009, Turlock, Calif. 95380.)

If you have syringes or needles, carry a note from your physician explaining why you need them. A physician's note for needles or syringes is almost always required for security reasons during flights and may be required on other forms of transportation or when you are driving across national boundaries. Let airline agents and screening personnel know *in advance* about any artificial joints or metal shoe inserts that may trigger detectors.

If you are planning to travel out of the country, find out what your health insurance will cover in terms of medical care in other countries. Additional, temporary coverage is sometimes available. Always purchase trip insurance for large, expensive trips, in case you have a serious flare-up and are unable to travel as scheduled.

Driving Tips

Stop the car frequently, and get out and stretch. This will help you avoid stiffness and soreness.

Rental cars often have such features as tiltable steering wheels, cruise control, and power steering. Rental cars with wide-angled rearview and sideview mirrors (helpful if you have arthritis in your neck), adjustable headrests, and auto aids such as padded steering wheels and right- and left-hand controls are also sometimes available.

In cold weather have someone else warm up the car before you get into it.

Lever aids that can be put on door and ignition keys help those who find it difficult to turn a key because of arthritis in the fingers.

Grab handles can be attached to the ridge of the roof to help you get in and out of the car.

Keep medications in the glove compartment rather than in the trunk so they will not be exposed to extreme changes in temperature.

Pack snacks and a beverage so you can take your medications on schedule. Set a wrist watch alarm or carry a very small folding travel alarm clock to remind you to take your medication.

Neck, back, and seat cushions in various styles and materials are available to support painful areas. Special seat-belt cushioning can be added to decrease shoulder discomfort.

When Traveling by Air

Notify the airline in advance of any special needs you have. Airline personnel can help you with your luggage and assist you in boarding and getting off the airplane. Airlines can often accommodate special diets.

Try to travel during light air traffic hours and the least busy weeks of the year. It's best to avoid crowds.

Never be embarrassed to ask for assistance. Do not hesitate to use the "pre-board" option.

If possible, find a flight that will deliver you to your destination without stopping in another city on the way, *especially if the flight involves changing planes*. If it isn't possible to book a nonstop flight, allow for adequate time between flights. Arrangements can be made to have a wheelchair or cart transport you and your luggage to the next departure area.

Request a bulkhead seat (the first row of seats) or an exit-row seat for more room. During flight, do simple range-of-motion exercises, particularly with your hips, knees, and feet, and when you are getting close to your destination.

Carry as little luggage as possible onto the airplane. Heavy luggage should be sent through normal airline luggage processes. Consider buying rolling carry-on hand bags, with long extendable handles, to minimize the stress on your hands and wrists.

If you are wheelchairbound, use the restroom before boarding the plane. Restrooms on board are often not easily accessible for someone in a wheelchair.

When planning a hotel or motel stop, call in advance to find out whether their facilities will meet your needs. If the facilities will make it difficult for you to maneuver or if they will force you to exert energy that you would rather save to use elsewhere, then you'll probably want to find someplace else to stay. Ask these questions:

· How close is the parking lot to my room?
· Where are the elevators in relationship to my room?
· Is it possible to book a room that has a bathroom with tub and toilet grab bars?
· (If you are in a wheelchair) Are there ramps, and are the doors to the room and bathroom wide enough to accommodate a wheelchair?

Pregnancy and Childbirth

Deciding whether or not to have children is a momentous decision for anyone. It is natural to have concerns about the health of a potential child, and most people think about this before or during pregnancy. Women of childbearing age who have RA will have specific questions about how their illness might affect their body and their unborn child.

Can I Become Pregnant?

Fertility is generally not affected by RA. During severe flare-ups, however, fertility may be temporarily lower in some individuals. But you should not count on this as a method of birth control, since it is not a failproof method.

How Will Pregnancy Affect My RA?

More than 75 percent of women see improvement in their RA during pregnancy. After delivery, most of them find that their arthritis returns to its prepregnancy level.

How Will My RA Affect My Unborn Child?

The health of the fetus and newborn infant does not appear to be affected adversely by RA, although this question has not been studied adequately for us to state unequivocally that this is so.

We do know that certain arthritis medications can compromise your baby's health. If you are considering getting pregnant or if you are sexually active and are not using birth control, you *must* discuss your medications with your physician. *This is important for men as well as women.* To be cleared completely out of your body, several arthritis medications need to be discontinued months or weeks before conception takes place or the child might be affected. Chapters 12 and 13 provide general recommendations about drugs, pregnancy, and breastfeeding, but your own doctor can best advise you on this subject.

Can I Breastfeed My Infant?

In most circumstances, breastfeeding is an option, although there is some new evidence that breastfeeding can increase the risk of postpartum flair in RA (Barrett, 2000). If a flare-up occurs, medications may be necessary to calm it. Medications, routine or for a flare-up, can be excreted in the breast milk, and breastfeeding is not recommended for women taking some RA medications. Please discuss breastfeeding with your doctor.

Will My Child Have RA?

After reading the discussion earlier in this book about the role of genes in the development of RA, you may be wondering whether this is a condition that will be passed on to your children. Remember, though, that genes tell only part of the story. We do not know exactly what triggers the development of RA. It is true that a person who has a close family member with RA or another autoimmune condition has a higher likelihood of developing RA than the general population. We do not feel that the small increased risk of passing on RA should influence a person's decision about childbearing. The vast majority of children born to a parent with RA do not develop the condition.

Will I Be Able to Care for My Baby?

This is perhaps the most difficult question. Caring for a baby requires a great deal of energy and stamina on the part of the caregiver. Performing frequent diaper changes and carrying around an extra 10 to 20 pounds can put a serious strain on tender joints. Feedings at two o'clock in the morning tire out even healthy parents. And, as we have discussed, joint stress, fatigue, and exhaustion can make arthritis and its symptoms worse.

You and your partner need to discuss these issues honestly with each other. You both need to be committed to creating and carrying out a plan that will allow the person with RA to get adequate rest. Putting aside extra funds for child care assistance is an excellent idea. Using disposable diapers will help, so that you don't have to manipulate diaper pins and wring out soiled diapers. You may want to invest in a carrier for holding the infant and get advice from an **occupational therapist** about how you can carry the baby while putting the least amount of stress on your joints. Plan ahead, and make certain that your plans include the toddler years.

Immunization for the Person with RA

Should I Get a Yearly Flu Shot?

Many physicians recommend yearly influenza, or "flu," vaccinations for people with RA. This is because RA is a chronic illness and because many people with RA take medications (**immunosuppressants, biologic response modifiers,** and **corticosteroids**) that can impair the body's ability to ward off an infection like the flu. The flu vaccination is generally safe and effective.

Are There Other Vaccinations That I May Want to Get?

Sometimes it is recommended that people with RA receive a vaccination against a form of pneumonia called *pneumococcal pneumonia.* This vaccination is called Pneumovax. You may want to discuss this vaccine with your doctor. If you do receive it, keep a written record of it in a safe place, so you can remember when and where you received it should you be asked about it in the future.

All other vaccines should be reviewed with your rheumatologist. Some "live" vaccines should not be given with some medications (see chapters 13 and 14).

RA in Children and Adolescents

Children and adolescents can develop a form of RA known as *juvenile rheumatoid arthritis* or, more commonly, *JRA*. Despite the similarity in names, this is a condition that is entirely different from the adult form. The term *JRA* stands for more than one condition; in fact, we know of at least three different types of JRA: *polyarticular onset JRA* (meaning many joints are affected), *pauciarticular JRA* (meaning a few joints are affected), and *systemic onset JRA* (meaning systems beyond the joints are affected). The different types of JRA are very dissimilar from each other in terms of the joints involved and the symptoms that occur.

Treatment of JRA is similar in some ways to the treatment of adult RA, but it is also different in many ways. For example, periodic eye examinations are required for some children with JRA, because asymptomatic eye problems can develop. Many of the medications used to treat adult RA are also used to treat JRA, but doses differ, and the medications sometimes cause side effects in children which they don't cause in adults. All medications and side effects should be discussed with the pediatrician or a pediatric **rheumatologist** (a specialist whose training differs from that of the adult rheumatologist in many instances).

Physical therapy and **occupational therapy** are even more important for children than for adults, since, unlike adults, children are still growing. In addition, children's joints are much more likely than adults' joints to freeze up and lose range of motion.

Also, JRA affects children emotionally and socially differently than RA affects adults, but the child's parents are generally more emotionally upset by the arthritis than the child is. Often the parents overprotect the child, emotionally and physically, preventing the child from experiencing the carefree time that kids need. If you are the parent of a child with JRA, we recommend that you

· avoid sheltering the child or preventing him or her from developing coping mechanisms that will be required long after you are no longer nearby to provide assistance;
· not make the child feel that he or she is "sick";
· discuss the specifics of the child's limitations with the rheumatologist before restricting the child's activities; and
· consult a pediatric counselor who is experienced in chronic disease and who can guide you and the child through behavior problems.

Your local chapter of the Arthritis Foundation can provide much more information about JRA than is provided in this book, which is intended for adults. The Arthritis Foundation can also give you information about the American Juvenile Arthritis Organization (AJAO), a national membership organization established by the Arthritis Foundation.

For More Information

A nonprofit corporation that combats health care fraud has a Web site: www.quackwatch.com.

The Food and Drug Administration has a Web site that provides information on how to spot health fraud: www.fda.gov/fdac/features/1999/699_fraud.html.

The Arthritis Foundation's Web site offers tips for car, air, train, and bus travel: www.arthritis.org/resources.

Reliable information on resources for the disabled traveler, including airlines, trains, buses, cruise lines, driving, and travel agents, can be found at: www.mossresourcenet.org.

Closing Thoughts

•

We leave you with ten thoughts and principles we think deserve special emphasis. For each person, life is a series of choices. We hope that the choices we recommend will nurture you and lead you to greater strength and a better place as you live with RA.

Choose hopefulness. Physicians and scientists have never been in a better position to understand RA and learn new ways of controlling this condition. The current discoveries and future possibilities are incredibly promising.

Choose knowledge. Learn as much as you can about RA. Find trusted advocates like the Arthritis Foundation and become an expert on your condition. This will empower you. This is the first step to self-efficacy—the ability to take control of your condition, both physically and mentally. Self-direction regarding your RA will flow over to other aspects of your life in a positive way.

Choose healthy habits. Get a good night's sleep. Limit alcohol. Do not smoke and avoid others who do. (Smoking has been shown to increase the severity of RA.) Give your body the fresh, clean air it deserves. Balance your activities. There is considerable evidence that a healthy life-style reduces the symptoms of RA.

Choose fitness and good nutrition. We have discussed nutrition in detail in this book. You'll have only one body. Listen to it. Respect it. Treat it as you would any prized possession.

Choose spirit. Feed your spirit as you would your body. Tap into your inner resources. Be open to self-discovery. Explore disciplines that help you open your spiritual self, such as meditation, yoga, tai chi, and religion, all practices that have stood the test of time.

Choose positivity. We have limited reserves of physical and emotional energy. Give yours to appreciation, understanding, and love. This will promote more energy. Use yours to learn new things or to exercise or to plan a lovely meal. Don't waste an ounce on anxiety, disappointment, guilt, or anger. These will empty the well and keep it dry. (Seek professional help if you are having trouble coping with anxiety, disappointment, guilt, or anger.)

Choose beauty. Surround yourself with things of beauty. Listen to great music. Take a walk in nature. Listen to the rain. Put on your favorite fragrance.

Choose joy. Resolve to bring joy and fun to your life. Like all things, even this takes a choice. Make this one, because you deserve it.

Choose communication. Choose to understand and to be understood. Make your needs known. Make sure you know what your loved ones need from you. You may be surprised to learn that the reality is different from what you expected and, possibly, easier to fulfill. Studies show that people with supportive relationships experience less pain.

Choose to simplify. We waste valuable resources on the unnecessary. Simplicity takes some discipline, because many things are competing for your time and attention. It is worth the energy to thoughtfully decide what is important and clear up the clutter in one's life. Only then can you make clear choices about your next step.

Glossary

•

Abduction: Movement of a part away from the midline of the body.

Adduction: Movement of a part toward the midline of the body.

Anemia: Low red blood cell count.

Antibodies: Protein that is formed by the body as a defense against a foreign substance (antigen) such as bacteria or viruses; also called immunoglobulins.

Antigen: Substance or material that is detected by the body as foreign.

Antioxidant: A vitamin, mineral, or other organic substance that helps prevent damaging effects of certain other substances in the body.

Arthrocentesis: Procedure to remove joint fluid with a needle; also called joint aspiration.

Arthroscope: Instrument used to view the inside of a joint by inserting a small scope through the skin.

Articulation: Another name for a joint.

Atrophy: Decreased size.

Autoantibodies: Antibodies that, although created by the body, cause the body to react against itself.

Autoimmunity: When the body inappropriately makes antibodies or immune reactions against its own tissues.

Biofeedback: Technique by which a person uses his or her own physiologic responses to achieve some control over the body's responses.

Biologic response modifier (BRM): New type of medication that is directed at very specific parts of the immune system.

Bone density test: Noninvasive diagnostic test that determines mineral density of the bone and can diagnose osteoporosis.

Bursa: Slippery sac that lies between tendons, muscles, and bones, promoting easy movement without friction.

Bursitis: Inflammation of the bursa.

Capsule: Fibrous enclosure surrounding a joint.

Cartilage: Tissue that covers the bone on each side of a joint.

Cell: Smallest living component of an organism.

273

Chondrocytes: Cartilage cell.

Chronic: Describing a condition or illness that may last months or years.

Clinical history: Description of symptoms.

Collagen: Structural protein important in the framework of cartilage and bone.

Collagenase: Enzyme that breaks down collagen and thus cartilage and bone.

Combination therapy: Use of two or more DMARDs at the same time.

Complete blood count (CBC): Estimate of the total number of red blood cells, white blood cells, and platelets in the body.

Connective tissue disease: Condition with inflammation involving the connective tissue (such as joints, skin, muscle). These disorders usually involve autoimmunity.

Corticosteroid: Strong anti-inflammatory medication; also called steroid or cortisone.

COX-2 (cyclo-oxygenase-2) inhibitors: New class of NSAID that causes less stomach side effects.

CRP (C reactive protein): Measurement of inflammation in the blood.

Cytokine: Chemical messenger produced by cells to govern the activity of other cells.

Dermatologist: Physician who specializes in care of and treatment of disorders of the skin.

Dietitian: Trained specialist who provides information about proper nutrition, special diets, and weight loss programs.

Differential diagnosis: List of possible diagnoses for a particular problem.

DMARD (disease-modifying antirheumatic drug): Medication used in the attempt to induce a remission of rheumatoid arthritis.

Effusion: Excessive accumulation of fluid.

Enzyme: Protein that can cause changes in other substances.

Episcleritis: Inflammation of the outer covering of the eye.

Erosion: Small hole in cartilage and bone which results from an inflamed joint lining (synovitis).

Erythrocyte: Red blood cell.

ESR (erythrocyte sedimentation rate or "sed rate"): Blood test that reflects the presence of inflammation in the body.

Extension: Straightening out of a joint.

Extra-articular: Symptom occurring outside the joint.

Felty's syndrome: Complication of rheumatoid arthritis consisting of an enlarged spleen and a low white blood cell count.

Flexion: Bending of a joint.

Gastritis: Inflammation of the stomach lining.

Gelling: Feeling of stiffness upon arising in the morning or after remaining in the same position for a long time.

Gluten: The major protein in wheat and some other whole grains.

Hand surgeon: A specialist in the medical and surgical treatment of hand problems; many doctors have special training and board certification in this subspecialty.

Hematocrit and hemoglobin: Measurements of red blood cells.

Hypertrophy: Increased size.

Imagery, visualization: Use of healing images to promote relaxation.

Immune system or immunity: Body's defense against foreign substances.

Immunosuppressant: A medication that suppresses the immune system and may thereby reduce symptoms of arthritis.

Inflammation: Complex reaction characterized by heat, swelling, redness, and pain.

Inflammatory arthritis: Arthritis caused by inflammation in the joints.

Interleukin-1 (IL-1): Cytokine known to cause inflammation and damage.

Joint effusion: Fluid in the joint.

Latex fixation: Test used to detect rheumatoid factor.

Leukotriene: Substance that is an extremely potent producer of inflammation.

Ligament: Cordlike structure that attaches bone to bone across joints, giving them stability.

Lymphocyte: Type of white blood cell involved in inflammation and infection fighting.

Macrophage: Type of cell that can engulf and destroy foreign substances.

Malaise: Vague feeling of illness.

Meditation: Discipline in which one directs or focuses the mind.

Neuropathy: Nerve problem leading to numbness or weakness.

Neutrophil: White blood cell involved in inflammation and infection fighting; also called polymorphonuclear cell or "poly."

Nodule: Small, painless lump that can occur over a bony prominence or a tendon.

NSAID (nonsteroidal anti-inflammatory drug): Medication that is used to decrease pain and inflammation.

Nurse: Trained health care provider who is knowledgeable about nursing procedures and medical science. There are several different kinds of nurses and nurse assistants: registered nurses, licensed practical nurses, nurse's aides, and nursing technicians.

Nutritionist: See **Dietitian.**

Occupational therapist: Person who teaches people how to perform their daily tasks in a fashion that accommodates their physical limitations. The occupational therapist may introduce adaptive equipment that allows independent living or make recommendations for changes in the home and workplace to improve functioning there. An occupational therapist is usually the specialist who designs wrist or hand splints and who teaches relaxation techniques and tips for conserving energy.

Ophthalmologist: Physician who is an eye specialist (differs from an optometrist, who measures vision, and an optician, who makes eyeglasses).

Orthopedic surgeon: Physician who specializes in surgery of the bones and joints.

Orthotics: Development and application of splints, braces, or other additional materials to improve function, decrease pain and inflammation, or to prevent deformity.

Orthotist: Person who fabricates specialized braces and corrective equipment used to improve the functioning of joints and muscles.

Osteoarthritis: Most common form of arthritis; also called degenerative joint disease.

Osteoporosis: Condition resulting from bone loss; it increases the risk of fracture.

Osteotomy: Surgical procedure that involves removing a piece of bone to realign the joint and reduce deformity.

Pannus: Inflamed synovial tissue when it moves along the cartilage and bone and breaks down joint tissue.

Pedorthist: Practitioner skilled in the design, manufacture, fit, and modification of prescription footwear and related devices for problem feet.

Pericardial effusion: Fluid around the heart.

Pericarditis: Inflammation of the covering of the heart (pericardium).

Pharmacist: Person trained in the preparation of medications. The pharmacist can provide information about drug side effects and drug interactions.

Physiatrist: Physician who is an expert in the field of exercise and rehabilitation. The physiatrist generally refers people with rheumatoid arthritis to the physical therapist or occupational therapist for a treatment program.

Physical therapist: Person trained to assess arthritis and organize an exercise program designed to meet an individual's needs. The physical therapist instructs people in methods of joint protection as well as in exercise programs designed to maintain joint mobility and muscle strength or to strengthen muscles and improve fitness and endurance without damaging the joints. A physical therapist also helps people to rehabilitate after joint surgery and to develop strategies of pain control, including heat therapy, cold therapy, hydrotherapy (water therapy), ultrasound, and electrotherapy, and instructs people in the proper use of walking aids.

Plasma cell: Type of white blood cell.

Plastic surgeon: A surgical specialist who operates on the skin as well as the underlying tendons, muscles, and other soft tissues.

Platelet: Blood cells responsible for clotting.

Pleural effusion: Fluid around the lungs.

Pleurisy: Inflammation of the lining around the lungs, resulting in pain with inspiration.

Pneumonitis: Inflammation of the lungs.

Podiatrist: Person who is trained solely in medical and surgical treatment of the feet. The podiatrist also makes recommendations about customized shoes and fabricates inserts or specialized orthotics to fit inside shoes to accommodate changes that have occurred in the feet.

Progressive relaxation: Relaxation program that focuses on successive regions of the body in a stepwise fashion.

Prostaglandin: Substance that produces and modifies inflammation.

Psychologist and psychiatrist: Mental health experts who can help people to cope with the challenges posed by having a chronic condition. A psychologist usually has either a master's or a doctorate degree, whereas a psychiatrist has the M.D. degree and can prescribe medications.

Remission: Period of time during which there is no evidence of active disease.

Rheumatoid factor: Special form of antibody which is found in 80 to 90 percent of people with rheumatoid arthritis.

Rheumatoid nodule: See **Nodule.**

Rheumatologist: A physician who is board certified in internal medicine and who specializes in the treatment of arthritis and other rheumatic diseases. Most rheumatologists are internists who have had special training in arthritis.

Rheumatology: Study of arthritis and related problems as well as the study of diseases of autoimmunity.

Scleritis: Inflammation of the white part of the eye, called the sclera.

Sepsis: Severe infection in which bacteria gets into the blood supply.

Social worker: Person educated and trained to provide information about support groups, counseling, and other local agencies and services. A social worker can also direct people to resources for help in solving problems related to finances, insurance, disability, job retraining, home care, housing, and legal issues.

Splint: Manufactured support used to stabilize and rest a given joint.

Subchondral bone: Bone found directly beneath (*sub*) the cartilage (*chondral*) in a joint.

Synovial cell: Cell in the joint lining.

Synovial fluid: Joint fluid.

Synovial joint: Joint that is freely movable, has a synovial lining, and is affected in rheumatoid arthritis; also called a diarthrodial joint.

Synovitis: Inflammation of the synovial lining.

Synovium: Joint lining; also called synovial membrane or synovial lining.

Systemic: Affecting more than one part of the body.

Tendinitis: Inflammation of a tendon.

Tendon: Structure that attaches muscle to bone; often surrounded by a tendon sheath.

Tenosynovitis: Inflammation of the tendon and surrounding joint lining.

Tissue: Body component such as cartilage, muscle, and bone.

Titer: Measurement that reflects the quantity of a substance present in blood.

Tumor necrosis factor (TNF): Cytokine known to cause inflammation.

Vasculitis: Inflammation of the blood vessels.

White blood cell: Cell involved in the complex functions of defense against infection and inflammation.

Bibliography

•

Barrett, J. 2000. "Breast-feeding and Postpartum Relapse in Women with Rheumatoid and Inflammatory Arthritis." *Arthritis and Rheumatism* 43 (May): 1010–15.

Barton-Wright, E. C., et al. 1963. "The Pantothenic Acid Metabolism of Rheumatoid Arthritis." *Lancet* 2:862–63.

Bernstein, H. N. 1983. "Ophthalmologic Considerations and Testing in Patients Receiving Long-term Antimalarial Therapy." *American Journal of Medicine* suppl. 1A (July 18): 25–34.

Brown, B. G., et al. 2001. "Simvastatin and Niacin, Antioxidant Vitamins, or the Combination for the Prevention of Coronary Disease." *New England Journal of Medicine* 345 (November 29): 1583–92.

Cohen, A., et al. 1964. "Bromelain Therapy in Rheumatoid Arthritis." *Pennsylvania Medical Journal* 67:27–30.

Comstock, G. W., et al. 1997. "Serum Concentrations of Alpha-tocopherol, Beta-carotene, and Retinol Preceding the Diagnosis of Rheumatoid Arthritis and Systemic Lupus Erythematosus." *Annals of the Rheumatic Diseases* 56 (May): 323–25.

Cutolo, M. 2000. "Sex Hormone Adjuvant Therapy in Rheumatoid Arthritis." *Rheumatic Disease Clinics of North America* 26 (November): 881–95.

Darlington, L. G. 2001. "Antioxidants and Fatty Acids in the Amelioration of Rheumatoid Arthritis and Related Disorders." *British Journal of Nutrition* 85 (March): 251–69.

Deluca, H. F., and M. L. Cantoma. 2001. "Vitamin D: Its Role and Uses in Immunology." *FASEB Journal* 15 (December): 2579–85.

DiSilvestro, R. A., et al. 1992. "Effects of Copper Supplementation on Ceruloplasmin and Copper-Zinc Superoxide Dismutase in Free-living Rheumatoid Arthritis Patients." *Journal of the American College of Nutrition* 11 (April): 177–80.

Enliven Panel. 2000. "RA and Intimacy." Wyeth-Ayerst Pharmaceuticals and Immunex Corporation.

Fairburn, K., et al. 1992. "Alpha-tocopherol, Lipids and Lipoproteins in Knee-joint Synovial Fluid and Serum from Patients with Inflammatory Joint Disease." *Clinical Science* 83:657–64.

Fisher, P., and D. L. Scott. 2001. "A Randomized Controlled Trial of Homeopathy in Rheumatoid Arthritis." *Rheumatology* 40 (September): 1052–55.

Fraser, D. A., et al. 2000. "Serum Levels of Interleukin-6 and Dehydroepiandosterone Sulphate in Response to Fasting or a Ketogenic Diet in Rheumatoid Arthritis." *Clinical and Experimental Rheumatology* 18 (May–June): 357–62.

General Practitioner Research Group. 1980. "Calcium Pantothenate in Arthritic Conditions." *Practitioner,* 208–11.

Grant, W. B. 2000. "The Role of Meat in the Expression of Rheumatoid Arthritis." *British Journal of Nutrition* 84 (November): 589–95.

Gray, R. G., and N. L. Gottlieb. 1985. "Adverse Reactions from Antirheumatic Drugs." *Rheumatoid Arthritis: Etiology, Diagnosis, Management.* Philadelphia: J. B. Lippincott.

Gutweniger, S., et al. 1999. "Body Image of Women with Rheumatoid Arthritis." *Clinical and Experimental Rheumatology* 17:413–17.

Hafstrom, I., et al. 2001. "A Vegan Diet Free of Gluten Improves the Signs and Symptoms of Rheumatoid Arthritis: The Effects on Arthritis Correlate with a Reduction in Antibodies to Food Antigens." *Rheumatology* 40 (October): 1175–79.

Hanninen, O., et al. 2000. "Antioxidants in Vegan Diet and Rheumatic Disorders." *Toxicology* 1555 (November): 45–53.

Hardin, J. G., and G. L. Longenecker. 1992. *Handbook of Drug Therapy in Rheumatic Disease: Pharmacology and Clinical Aspects.* Boston: Little, Brown.

Harris, E. D., Jr. 1990. "Rheumatoid Arthritis: Pathophysiology and Implications for Therapy." *New England Journal of Medicine* 322 (May 3): 1277–89.

Haslock, I., et al. 1994. "Measuring the Effects of Yoga in Rheumatoid Arthritis." *British Journal of Rheumatology* 33 (August): 787–88.

Heinle, K., et al. 1997. [Selenium Concentration in Erythrocytes of Patients with Rheumatoid Arthritis: Clinical and Laboratory Chemistry Infection Markers during Administration of Selenium] *Medizinische Klinik* 92, suppl. 3 (September): 29–31. (In German.)

Helmy, M., et al. 2001. "Antioxidants as Adjuvant Therapy in Rheumatoid Arthritis: A Preliminary Study." *Arzneimittelforschung* 51:293–98. (In English.)

Horstman, J. 1999. *The Arthritis Foundation's Guide to Alternative Therapies.* Atlanta: Arthritis Foundation.

Jordan, J. M., et al. 2000. "Self-reported Arthritis-related Disruptions in

Sleep and Daily Life and the Use of Medical, Complementary, and Self-care Strategies for Arthritis: The National Survey of Self-care and Aging." *Archives of Family Medicine* 9 (February): 143–49.

Kajanachumpol, S., et al. 2000. "Levels of Plasma Lipid Peroxide Products and Antioxidant Status in Rheumatoid Arthritis." *Southeast Asian Journal of Tropical Medicine and Public Health* 31 (June): 335–38.

Kinlen, L. J. 1985. "Incidence of Cancer in Rheumatoid Arthritis and Other Disorders after Immunosuppressive Treatment." *American Journal of Medicine* 78, suppl. 1A:44–49.

Kirsteins, A. E., et al. 1991. "Evaluating the Safety and Potential Use of a Weight-bearing Exercise, Tai-Chi Chuan, for Rheumatoid Arthritis Patients." *American Journal of Physical Medicine and Rehabilitation* 70 (June): 136–41.

Kjeldsen-Kragh, J. 1999. "Rheumatoid Arthritis Treated with Vegetarian Diets." *American Journal of Clinical Nutrition* 70 (September): 594s–660s.

Kjeldsen-Kragh, J., et al. 1991. "Controlled Trial of Fasting and One-Year Vegetarian Diet in Rheumatoid Arthritis." *Lancet* 338:899–902.

Kjeldsen-Kragh, J., et al. 1995a. "Changes in Laboratory Variables in Rheumatoid Arthritis Patients during a Trial of Fasting and One-Year Vegetarian Diet." *Scandinavian Journal of Rheumatology* 24:85–93.

Kjeldsen-Kragh, J., et al. 1995b. "Decrease in Anti-*Proteus mirabilis* but Not Anti-*Escherichia coli* Antibody Levels in Rheumatoid Arthritis." *Annals of the Rheumatic Diseases* 54:221–24.

Knekt, P., et al. 2000. "Serum Selenium, Serum Alpha-tocopherol, and the Risk of Rheumatoid Arthritis." *Epidemiology* 11:402–5.

Kremer, J. M. 2000. "N-3 Fatty Acid Supplements in Rheumatoid Arthritis." *American Journal of Clinical Nutrition* (January): 349s–351s.

Levinski, W. K., and J. Lansbury. 1951. "An Attempt to Transmit Rheumatoid Arthritis to Humans." *Proceedings of the Society of Experimental Biology and Medicine* 78.

Linos, A., et al. 1999. "Dietary Factors in Relation to Rheumatoid Arthritis: A Role for Olive Oil and Cooked Vegetables?" *American Journal of Clinical Nutrition* 70 (December): 1077–82.

Lucas, C. P., et al. 1981. "Dietary Fat Aggravates Active Rheumatoid Arthritis." *Clinical Research* 29:754A.

Maksymowych, W., and A. S. Russel. 1987. "Antimalarial in Rheumatology: Efficacy and Safety." *Seminars in Arthritis and Rheumatism* 18 (February): 206–21.

McNeal, R. L. 1990. "Aquatic Therapy for Patients with Rheumatic Disease." *Rheumatic Disease Clinics of North America* 16 (November): 915–29.

Matthews, D. A., et al. 2000. "Effects of Intercessory Prayer on Patients with Rheumatoid Arthritis." *Southern Medical Journal* 93:1177–86.

Melzack, R., and P. Wall. 1983. *The Challenge of Pain*. New York: Basic Books.

Mikuls, T. R., et al. 2002. "Coffee, Tea, and Caffeine Consumption and the Risk of Rheumatoid Arthritis: Results from the Iowa Women's Health Study." *Arthritis and Rheumatism* 46: 83–91.

Minor, M. A., and N. E. Lane. 1996. "Recreational Exercise in Arthritis." *Rheumatic Disease Clinics of North America* 22 (August): 563–77.

Muller, H., et al. 2001. "Fasting Followed by Vegetarian Diet in Patients with Rheumatoid Arthritis." *Scandinavian Journal of Rheumatology* 30:1–10.

Panush, R. S., ed. 2000. "Complementary and Alternative Therapies for Rheumatic Diseases: I. and II." *Rheumatic Disease Clinics of North America* (February).

Peretz, A., et al. 2001. "Selenium Supplementation in Rheumatoid Arthritis Investigated in a Double-blind, Placebo-controlled Trial." *Scandinavian Journal of Rheumatology* 30:208–12.

Roubenoff, R., et al. 1997. "Abnormal Homocysteine Metabolism in Rheumatoid Arthritis." *Arthritis and Rheumatism* 40:718–22.

Scammell, H. 1998. *The New Arthritis Breakthrough*. New York: M. Evans.

Social Security Administration. 2001. *2001 Red Book on Employment Support: A Summary Guide to Employment Support Available to People with Disabilities under the Social Security Disability Insurance and Supplemental Security Income Programs* (January).

Stafford, L., et al. 2000. "Androgen Deficiency and Bone Mineral Density in Men with Rheumatoid Arthritis." *Journal of Rheumatology* 27 (December): 2786–90.

Stone, J., et al. 1997. "Inadequate Calcium, Folic Acid, Vitamin E, Zinc and Selenium Intake in Rheumatoid Arthritis Patients: Results of a Dietary Survey." *Seminars in Arthritis and Rheumatism* 27:180–85.

Tarp, U. 1995. "Selenium in Rheumatoid Arthritis: A Review." *Analyst* 3:877–81.

Tilley, B. C., et al. 1995. "Minocycline in Rheumatoid Arthritis: A 48-Week, Double-Blind, Placebo-Controlled Trial." *Annals of Internal Medicine* 122:81–89.

Travers, R. L., et al. 1990. "Boron and Arthritis: The Results of a Double-blind Pilot Study." *Journal of Nutritional Medicine*, 127–32.

U.S. Department of Health and Human Services. 1995. *Nutrition and Your Health: Dietary Guidelines for Americans*. 4th ed.

Walker, W. R., and D. M. Keats. 1976. "An Investigation of the Therapeutic Value of the Copper Bracelet: Dermal Assimilation of Copper in Arthritic/Rheumatoid Conditions." *Agents Actions* 6:454–59.

Wolfe, F. 2000. "The Effect of Smoking on Clinical, Laboratory, and Radiographic Status in Rheumatoid Arthritis." *Journal of Rheumatology* 27 (March): 630–37.

Zurier, R. B., et al. 1996. "Gamma-Linolenic Acid Treatment of Rheumatoid Arthritis: A Randomized, Placebo-controlled Trial." *Arthritis and Rheumatism* 39 (November): 1808–17.

Index

•